Author's note

I wrote most everything in this story while it was happening to me, moment by moment, because in the absence of anything to hold onto, I was desperate to keep events from overwhelming me. Taking notes felt like a way to slow things down enough for my brain to try to process what was going on. After awhile I had a gigantic pile of notes, which I stuck away in a drawer in the irrational hope that by burying them I could somehow bury all that they spoke about. But in short order I was back writing notes once more, this time in the form of emails to friends and family, hoping I could slow them down from barraging me with questions. Those emails evidently got forwarded on to people I'd never met, which I only learned about when several of those strangers wrote to me and said, essentially: "I don't know you, and I don't know quite how to say this, but I've really enjoyed reading about all your troubles. You should share this with other people."

As you'll see, the story is written in the present tense. Had this book originated as a memoir, I suppose I'd have used the past tense, but I didn't just wake up one day and say: "Hmm, that was a pretty crazy time in my life. I should write a book about it." Instead I made a deal with myself that if I made it through to the end I'd pull out the old pile of notes and see if there was anything worth sparing from an eternity in the drawer. As I began to read the notes, I felt as if I were right there again, and although it wasn't easy to revisit a lot of those emotions, I couldn't believe how many details I would have forgotten had I never written them down.

They say adversity introduces a man to himself. If that's true, then it's been fairly awful getting to know me. But in a strange way, kind of wonderful too. Which brings me to a point about *schadenfreude*.

At this point the gloves are off. They always have been. So feel free to enjoy my travails, and to laugh as I slip on one banana peel after another. I'm happy to be around to watch you laugh, believe me.

NOW IT'S FUNNY:

How I Survived Cancer, Divorce and Other Looming Disasters.

Michael Solomon

ISBN: 1463749554
ISBN-13: 9781463749552
Library of Congress Control Number: 2011918294
CreateSpace, North Charleston, SC

Table of Contents

"Through humor, you can soften some of the worst blows that life delivers. And once you find laughter, no matter how painful your situation might be, *you can survive it.*"

-Bill Cosby

Faust

A light rain is falling. Traffic along the narrow, newly paved road is slow and heavy. A python of automobiles snakes behind the black hearse limousine at the front of the procession. Inside the trailing vehicles, several fetchingly dressed, tormented women fight back tears, each of them asking themselves the same question: " Why did I make such poor choices in my life? Why didn't I seize happiness when it was within my grasp? What would I give just to have another moment with him, my true love, the only man I've ever really loved?" Seated next to these lovely women are several individuals involved in movie financing. Their riches have been thoroughly squandered. Their careers have been destroyed by silly movies that no one ever came to see. They are here today only to pay tribute to what could have been. To the dreams they once held for themselves. To the talent they saw yet failed to embrace. Their sorrow is overwhelming and painful. Physically and emotionally painful.

Welcome to my funeral.

It is a virtual Who's Who of people who have acted badly toward me. Women who left me for other men, actors who refused to read my screenplays, even my junior year college professor who gave me a C plus on my thesis paper about Jim Morrison and The Doors because I'd handwritten it instead of typing it. I wasn't expecting him to show up today, but it turns out his teaching career since I graduated has been idiotic and meaningless. I hear he's considering suicide once the funeral is over.

I usually go to my funeral when I'm in the shower, though I once attended it only seconds after a particularly unsatisfying lovemaking session. I'm sorry. My mind drifts a lot and I can't always control when it will take me away from whatever it is that I should be thinking about, though what exactly a person *should* be thinking about after an encounter like that is a bit of a mystery to me anyway. Celibacy? At least I wasn't thinking about the funeral of another woman.

I'm a bit twisted. I admit it. But the older I get, the more I feel like I'm not alone in my twisted state. I think people get more twisted as they age, and even though that would never actually allow for other formerly untwisted people to fully catch up with me, it would at least explain why I feel I've got company now. We've all crossed the same threshold, just at different times. I recognize this disparity from high school. Back in high school, you wouldn't think of dating someone in junior high (okay, maybe....I don't know about you, but I was pretty desperate). But by the time you reach thirty, the entire stigma about dating someone four years younger has vanished. This sort of process continues until at around fifty you might actually find yourself considering dating someone still in high school. Apply this form of attrition to twistedness, and you'll see that the fairly normal kids I knew when I was younger are now kind of screwed up too. Just like me.

I knew a guy in college, Matt, who wanted to get over his fear of death. I went to college at the University of California, Santa Barbara, and I can't say for sure if it was all the dope we smoked or just our youthfulness, but none of us thought it strange that a person would wake up one day, like Matt did, and decide that his fear of death was a pressing matter that required immediate and direct action.

Matt went out and got a job at a funeral home. He had the two qualifications necessary for the job; he was strong and he had a valid driver's license. Whenever the funeral home got a call about a new client, they sent Matt out in their hearse to pick up the body. Usually the bodies were still warm, and the mourners were still gathered around the bedside crying.

Matt lasted a week. Not because he couldn't handle the morbidity. Not because he couldn't handle the sadness. He quit because he was becoming even more afraid of death than before. Being close to death didn't bring any spiritual understanding, because it wasn't *his* death, it was always somebody else's. And there was no way to ask them for any insight. This inability to communicate made him feel even further from the truths he sought to learn.

Let's face it, life is absurdly short. Science says that evolution prefers us to live long enough to raise our children to the point of independence, after which we become expendable. We begin to deteriorate. Eventually we die. Evolution doesn't care about us having a productive retirement, or writing the novel we always wanted to write, or going back to school to get our master's degree.

Our fear of death is a fear of the loneliness of going wherever we go by ourselves. There are no loved ones to come with us and provide security. I know some people are afraid they'll go to Hell and burn, but these folks....I mean, come on....no one has ever in history returned from Hell to prove that it exists, which means it is as likely to be an inferno run by the Devil as it is to be a rubber factory, with a blackboard, where everyone spends eternity writing the word "Oberammergau" in purple chalk.

Evolution has programmed us to survive by avoiding death. After a while, it becomes a hard habit to break. We deny that death is really in the cards for us. I think what we truly fear is regret. The more I live, the more I feel that shame and regret, or more accurately the avoidance of shame and regret are the engines driving most human beings.

There's an old joke about a Jewish kid who goes to his father and asks: "Dad, can I borrow five dollars?" and his father says: "Four dollars? What do you need three dollars for?" To me this paradigm is emblematic of our struggle for longevity. We want to live forever, but the world is bent on getting rid of us.

Let me just come right out with it. Something really weird happened to me. Several weird things actually. Some by choice, others by accident. Nothing involving a kitchen utensil, luckily, but still an unusual confluence of unexpected changes in my life that lifted me off my feet, kicked me in the proverbial behind, and frequently left me groveling in despair and uncertainty. Not only did I revisit my funeral fantasy in my mind, I actually thought that I would be attending in person. It's been a hell of time. A time full of "big" thoughts. A time full of close calls. A time set in motion by the discovery that I did not have colon cancer. By the way, I never thought I had colon cancer. The only reason I even bothered to check is that in 1975 my grandfather the tailor died of colon cancer. My father -- his son and a bit of a hypochondriac -- had his first colonoscopy 17 years later, when he was fifty-eight years old. My father's doctor discovered several large polyps, or pre-cancerous growths, in his colon, which he subsequently removed with a colonoscope. A colonoscope is a long flexible metal tube that travels up your rear end and through your digestive tract. It has a camera and a surgical device that can cut out unwanted growths. My father subsequently called his two sisters and told them to have the same test done. One of them, my aunt in Hawaii, was told by her doctor that she only needed to have a sigmoidoscope done. The sigmoidoscope only travels partway up the colon, thus decreasing the risk of any tearing of the bowel walls.

Unfortunately for my aunt, her doctor was wrong. The sigmoidoscope test failed to reveal the colon cancer growing further up inside of her, and she wound up having to have surgery, chemotherapy and radiation because the cancer broke through the wall of her stomach. Luckily she survived.

Since then, my father has been hounding me and my siblings to have a colonoscopy done when we turned forty. He reminded me of it on the day of my fortieth birthday. The day after too. I've never imagined my father at my funeral, but if I did, I'm sure he'd be finding a way to tie whatever had caused my untimely death into my failure to have a colonoscopy done. He's really good at that sort of thing.

So one day, I find myself hanging out in my friend Steven's car. He's a pediatrician and a really decent guy. He's from South Africa and he dragged me along to Botswana a few summers ago on what turned out to be a rugged and superlative safari. We bought dope from Bushmen who buried their stashes in the sands of their front lawns, a.k.a. the Kalahari desert. Scratch that: for the purposes of propriety, let's just say that I bought the dope, okay?

Anyway, Steven and I are parked outside my apartment on Bleecker Street, using marijuana to try to conjure up our fond memories of the Africa trip. The farther away we get from the trip, the more need we feel to conjure like this. It's sort of a vicious cycle: we're getting older and more forgetful, so we smoke dope to get into a mental state where we can remember better, only to emerge with a memory further depleted by the dope we just smoked. I believe this is called the law of diminishing returns.

I mention to Steven that my father's been sweating me non-stop about going to have a colonoscopy because of the history of colon cancer in my family (his side of course, the fucker!). He says: "Who's your doctor?" and I say, "I don't have one." Steven says: "Yes you do. His name is Faust. Dr. Michael Faust. He's great. Everyone in my practice goes to him and now you're going too."

I say okay, but of course I'm thinking "Faust?" What kind of name is that for a doctor? Why not send me to Dr. Frankenstein while you're at it?

A few days later I call Faust and set up an appointment. I've passed my fortieth birthday, and haven't seen a general practitioner since a case of genital warts 15 years ago. Don't ask. I had them removed by a Jewish doctor named Plotnik, who insisted on discussing her strong belief in the cause of West Bank settlers in Israel. I accidentally let slip that I was in love with a Lebanese woman, which is not exactly the thing you want to share with a radical Jew burning warts off your penis. I tried to finesse the situation by assuring Plotnik that it was I who had contracted the warts, possibly even from a Jewish former girlfriend, rather than my current love (a.k.a. the enemy) but her heart only seemed to harden as she administered the painful cleansing.

I go to my appointment with Faust and he does all the tests. He says: "There's nothing wrong with you." I say: "I know." He says: "All you guys, you turn forty and you think you need to come in and do a work up." I say: "It's my old man, Dr. Faust. He keeps telling me I need a colonoscopy." Faust tells me to dress and meet him in his office.

He says that normally he wouldn't recommend a colonoscopy before age 50, but given my family history, he feels it would be prudent to do the test now, and then come back in another 5 or 10 years and do it again. He hands me a chart about risk versus frequency of testing, and then, almost as an afterthought, he writes me a prescription for a chest X-ray and says: "You should get a chest X-ray too."

From then on, I start delaying the colonoscopy appointment (the test itself, in which a sort of seeing-eye router takes a fantastic voyage through your intestines is not as horrid as it sounds. What's rough is the day before, when you fast and flush yourself with enough laxative to turn your insides into a *Mister Clean* commercial). I deposit the chest X-ray prescription on my desk at the office. It's a place where documents tend to lose meaning by sitting around and being looked at and then ignored so often. I'm the type of person who doesn't have a place to keep a chest X-ray prescription. I keep it on my desk so that it will become an irritant until I eventually surrender and put it to its proper use.

Faust calls me a couple of days later to say that the blood work came back from my check-up and my cholesterol is kind of high. "It's not alarming," he says "but you need to watch it. If it were alarming I'd be talking about prescribing medicine, but I'm not." He gives me my results – I can't even remember them – but one is a total cholesterol number and the other is a "bad" cholesterol number. I instantly flash on my father's best friend Bob. I remember him once boasting to my Dad that his cholesterol was some good low number or other and I thought: "This is aging. This is what happens from now on. You live longer but you spend those extra years talking about your cholesterol."

So I try to cool it on red meat and eggs and I struggle mightily to limit my chocolate intake. This lasts for three days. I discuss my predicament with Steven, at another conjuring session, and he laughs at my new lower cholesterol diet, saying that in all likelihood I'll have my cholesterol re-checked in a few months and it'll be even higher.

The real joke, he says, is that you ruin the best years of your life so you can live longer on the back end. More time to schlep around in your walker, unable to breathe, with a limp penis and a regimen of pills to take.

Nonetheless, or rather, despite that I agree with Steven I spend a few more weeks watching my intake. But a skim cappuccino in the morning quickly becomes a problem (my wife wants whole milk, I'd have to steam two types of milk separately, so forget it) and I learn that red wine lowers your cholesterol, so I start to drink it more regularly (to wash down the paté, for example). I stopped smoking six years ago after twenty years of huffing so it's particularly hard to restrict my one remaining pleasure -- food.

A couple of months go by. I am really not up for this colonoscopy. Instead, one afternoon, I pick up the prescription from my desk for the chest X-ray and dutifully set up an appointment. I'm thinking this may get me in the mood for the colonoscopy, and I congratulate myself on taking an active interest in my health.

I go for the chest X-ray. It takes all of five minutes. They send it off to Faust, he doesn't call me or anything, so now I'm just back to my cholesterol dilemma and the colonoscopy I still haven't had.

Dino

A week later I'm lying on the couch at home and the phone rings. The caller ID says "Faust, Michael." It's 9 o'clock at night. The call about cholesterol had come to my office so I make a quick assumption ("I'm dying") then answer the phone.

"Hello Michael. It's Doctor Faust."

"Oh hi," I say, thinking it impolite to tell him that I already know who it is from caller ID. I'm guessing it's about the chest X-ray.

"I've got your chest X-ray here," ("At home?! I'm definitely dying now!"). The radiologist saw something very small, it's probably old and nothing to worry about."

"Nothing alarming," I posit.

"No. Not alarming."

I say: "What's with you and the not-alarming stuff?" First, it's my not-alarming cholesterol, then it's my not-alarming this thing…"

We share a laugh and I sense that it really is not alarming.

He says he thinks it may be something called an old granuloma, and since I used to be a smoker, I should have a CT scan done just to be safe. He says: "Don't worry, but do this."

The next morning I make the appointment for the following Friday.

What hits me is that the distant bliss of my cigarette smoking life has suddenly returned as a hydra rearing its ugly (but tiny!) head. I have trouble wrapping my brain around any damage to my lung, old or new, caused by smoking. When you quit you start to develop a mental picture of utopian lungs, almost like a park, with fields of long cilia flowing in the breeze and butterflies rising up to a cloudless blue sky. It's said your lungs need seven years to regenerate and so I, in year six, imagine just a bit of excess litter on the ground, like an overfilled garbage canister after a public concert. Someone will be along in year seven to clean it up.

I've always believed life is full of cruel irony. When I went for the chest X-ray, I thought to myself "Isn't this the type of 'routine' test you always hear about that then uncovers something truly awful?"

I call Steven and he reassures me it's probably nothing. I've already developed a joke, telling my wife that what I have is actually an Indian dish called granuloma pakora. I look up granuloma disease on the Internet and find there is an entire organization of granuloma disease sufferers but it's not what I have at all - it's some full-blown, terrible disease. I decide to purge the Internet from my medical life.

Meantime by coincidence, I've made arrangements for my wife, a truly hardened smoker, to see some Russian nut job in Massachusetts who apparently treats the worst of the worst with extraordinary success. Here's where the irony kicks in- I tell my wife that I'll probably be the one to wind up with lung cancer even though *I* quit.

The Russian treats people who continue to smoke through holes in their trachea. The Russian treats people who've already had a lung removed. His therapy takes two hours - one time, two hours. I ask the receptionist on the phone what exactly he does and she says in matter of fact Russian-accented English: "*Hye* uses bio-energy. *Hye* traces back your urge to *smyoke* and *remyoves* it." I'd been reassuring my wife that the Russian wasn't a quack, so I don't share this tidbit of info with her. When I tell her about the appointment, I figure anything's worth a try with her. Once, when she became pregnant with our son, she tried the nicotine patch, but this just led to her smoking *and* wearing the patch. I told her she needed to wait until they invent a patch you wear over your mouth. Failing that, why not give this loopy Russian a try?

On Friday I get the CT scan, which is also known as a CAT scan. I'm led into a room containing a giant, donut-shaped machine not unlike an MRI tube, only too short to entomb you. Imagine passing through a Lifesaver on your back; that's your CAT scan machine. Now imagine lying on a conveyor belt inside an excruciatingly narrow mineshaft; that's more what an MRI is like.

I lay down on a moving tray, a laser light goes on as something mechanical-sounding swirls through the donut at high speed, and I'm slowly conveyed in and out of the donut while some sort of laser takes pictures of me. I know it's a laser because a sign tells me not to stare at it. The photo session lasts for five minutes. The specialist asks me why I'm there. I tell him I have a possible old granuloma in my left lung, hilar area (that's what the prescription says) and he says "Smoker?" I say: "Ex" and briefly I feel I'd like to throttle him. I know he said "smoker" but it felt and sounded like "idiot." At the end of the scan he gives me a look that I decide not to read much into because I don't know if he has seen any results on all the high-tech screens in his little protective chamber. (Later I learn that my hunch was right, he was just a jerk giving me a look; he hadn't seen any test results yet).

About five hours later, I'm with my six-year-old son Luke at his occupational therapy appointment and my cell phone rings. It's Faust, but he must be calling me from the office because my display says "caller ID blocked." He says "Michael. I received the results of the CAT scan. The issue is..."

Right then I know something's wrong. What issue? I thought there was no issue. But actually I'm calmer than this and I just listen.

He says the granuloma turned out to be nothing. A false positive. My left lung is fine. But now, on the other lung, my right lung, they've found something three centimeters in diameter (a little bit bigger than an inch). Not only that, they've seen something on my liver too, though it's probably not a tumor but rather some sort of clogged blood vessel related blah, blah, blah.

At this point, of course, I've lost my concentration. I'm sure I just heard the word "tumor." Faust says: "I even asked the radiologist 'are you sure you have the right patient?' But he said he was sure."

Damn, that seemed like the obvious explanation. El Pricko at the lab mixed me up with someone else. Maybe they do have the wrong guy! I instantly flash on an episode of the Flintstones where Fred and Dino's X-rays got mixed up. The doctor ordered Barney to keep Fred up all night or else. I can still see Fred's exhausted face, his eyes held open by toothpicks, his lower lip distended from Barney pulling it out and pouring endless pots of coffee into his mouth to keep him awake. All of this in a bowling alley.

Faust says he's concerned, in a way that means he's REALLY concerned. I'm thinking: "Did I just find out I have lung cancer?" They don't just come out and say: "You have lung cancer." They describe things and dimensions and locations and from these various ellipses you have to draw the picture yourself.

Faust says he wants me to have a pulmonary specialist "settle this" and he tells me we also need to "work up" the liver thing. Faust is a gastroenterologist, so I assume the liver problem slides neatly into his domain.

I hang up and look over at my son. I know instantly that this, that he, is the only loss I can not bear to think about. I'm deeply involved in his life and not at all prepared to take leave of it. I am bewildered. That I have no symptoms of any of this, only contributes to my puzzlement. I struggle to remember what Faust said about my liver and all I can recall is blood vessels something or other and even this I believe was a hopeful stab on his part to make sense of a mystery. For one idiotic second, I actually feel angry that they looked at my other lung and my liver – as though it were a violation of my privacy. It is hard to know what to do. A voice inside me is reminding me that I'm forty years old and nowhere near any sort of modern life expectancy. I once read in a work of fiction that lung cancer is basically a death sentence, although I more recently read a non-fiction account of a woman who is fourteen years into lung cancer survival, which would still only get me to 54, while my son would be 19. Plus this woman had part of her lung removed in surgery.

I decide that even though I want to tell someone, if not everybody, I'm gonna keep my mouth shut until I get something a bit more concrete. The specter of pity from my friends and family is horrifying. And already I feel ridiculous, like some two-bit stockbroker caught trading crummy insider information for a meager profit. For all the smoking I did in nearly 20 years, there was little satisfaction, save for the daily ritual of putting my craving to rest every half hour or so. Both my parents smoked, though ironically they quit because my sister and I so despised their smoking that we drove them crazy; badgering them, begging them, even opening up an entire carton of Tareytons and drawing rings halfway up 200 cigarettes to indicate the point at which, according to the American Cancer Society ad running at the time, they ought to put their cigarettes out, to reduce the danger of heart disease and lung cancer. The more irony I uncover in my story, the more frightened I am that I've become the protagonist of a cruel and bitter joke.

I decide I'll try to hold on until Wednesday, the day of my appointment with the pulmonary specialist. I relegate the liver to the town of Denialsville, especially because I don't see Faust until Thursday and by then, I may know I'm dying of something else. I realize that I may be setting my own irony trap as in: "wouldn't it be ironic if I died from the less serious whatever-is-wrong-with-my-liver thing?" But I decide this is a working plan and I'm gonna stick with it.

I drop off Luke and head back for a quick half hour at the office. I walk in and the two young women who work for me – Elena and Stephanie - look mortified. Elena says: "Did the doctor find you?" He hadn't of course revealed anything when he called my office, but his needing to know my cell phone number right away was enough of a tip off for them. I don't feel up to lying so I tell them what I know and say that really, still, I don't know anything. They start telling me there are a thousand factors which could cause this to add up to nothing; misdiagnosis, just some benign growth, and so on, and now I'm really sure I'm not gonna tell anyone else what's going on. It's so easy to believe that what someone else has is nothing, but good luck convincing *them* of that. This feels like a bad trip I don't want to be talked down from. I just want to see what is knowable and what my options are. Having two "issues," a liver issue and a lung issue, feels like it automatically rules out the realm of denial. Christ, whatever it is, I must have *something!*

A few hours later I'm at my marriage counselor's office with my wife. On the day we were married, a monstrous thunderstorm drenched the New York area, building eventually into a hailstorm. These types of summer weather events are not all that unusual, and probably mean very little symbolically, unless like me, you are a Jew marrying a Muslim, and unless your mother-in-law, like mine, is in the back seat of your car on the way to the ceremony pointing up to the heavens and proclaiming: "You see what God thinks of this wedding?!" All of a sudden the weather takes on a whole new significance. Then when things aren't going so well in your marriage, say about ten years later, you find that the meteorological episodes of that long ago summer tend to rise up from your memory to haunt you.

Luckily, the story of our wedding came to a happy conclusion. About fifteen minutes before it was scheduled to start, on a rented ferry boat no less, the hail stopped, the rain subsided, and the clouds suddenly bolted off towards the sunset, leaving us with a beautiful summer sky and a canopy of stars under which to tie the knot.

Our marriage, unfortunately, hasn't fared as well. We nearly split up a couple of years ago, seemed to get back on a more engaged and happy track, then fell back into a life marked more by separateness than by togetherness. And so tonight I decide that since my marriage has enough problems to fill the agenda, this won't be where I drop the bomb about my health and possible newfound lack of it. At the end of an hour, my wife and I are practically in a fight. So much for the benefits of counseling.

I'm up for a good part of the night processing my despair over my marriage and now, the lung thing. Two days pass and we learn that our babysitter, who went in to have cysts removed from her ovaries, is actually pregnant. She was worried about possibly losing an ovary as a result of surgery, and now not only are they putting off the surgery, her other ovary has obviously been working overtime. The pregnancy is great news and a hell of a lot better than the option of having her ovaries removed. "Maybe something like that will happen to me," I think. "Maybe I'm just pregnant."

Sunday night I sit my wife down and tell her the news about me. I say: "Do you remember the CAT scan I had to do?" and she says "Oh no!" She is stricken but she's good at denial. She tells me several times: "I'm sure you have nothing." She's trying to be encouraging but unfortunately I know what the score is at this point. The more we look, the more evidence there seems to be of trouble. She offers to come to Garay's office, the pulmonary specialist, but I say I want to go myself.

My appointment is at 3:30. I decide to pick up my films – the X-ray and the CT scan – after I drop Luke off at school. I take him to school every morning, and it feels especially important to me not to break from my rituals now. By 10 AM I'm back in my office with the films. I open the manila envelope and look at some of the pictures. I say to the girls: "It's my body. Even though I'm sure I can't tell anything from the pictures, I'm going to look anyway." I'm like the guy buying a car who kicks the tires because he's seen other people kicking the tires, even though he has no idea what this kicking is supposed to prove. I open the folder and look at some of the pictures.

The chest X-ray is totally illegible to me; I certainly don't see any huge blocks anywhere. The CAT scan is a series of 50 or so images, each looking like two lungs, although I have no clue as to their orientation, nor can I decipher anything from them. I then spy the typed radiologist's report and read it. When I'm done I say simply: "I'm fucked". I see panic in the girls' eyes so I then make a lame attempt at denying what I just so forcefully declared.

The report begins: "Dear Doctor: Computed axial tomography (CAT) of the chest."

It then lists a lot of things like tissues and arches as "unremarkable" or "well mineralized" until it says "evaluation of the lung parenchyma reveals a mass in the right middle lobe extending to the right pericardial border. This appears quite medial in position and measures approximately 3 cm in maximum diameter. Suggestion of an air bronchogram within this mass is identified. In view of the patient's lack of clinical symptoms, this is suspicious for malignancy possibly representing an alveolar cell carcinoma. Further evaluation is advised."

Wait a minute.

I read this last bit again. The conjecture that no symptoms may indicate a malignancy feels like a horrific betrayal. I'm fine ergo I'm dead?! Thinking it can't get worse, I go on. Blah, blah, blah, no adenopathy of right hilar (what I originally went in for). Blah, blah, and then "However, a 5 cm ill-defined mass is noted in the posterior aspect of the right lobe of the liver, low density and configuration." The liver thing. "Although this may represent benign lesion such as hemangioma, the possibility of metastasis cannot be excluded."

Metastasized cancer, I'm pretty sure, is cancer that has so thoroughly spread and infiltrated the body that treatment discussions simply turn to ways to make the doomed patient comfortable in the last days of their life. Synonyms for metastasis could include terminal, fatal or incurable. Later on, I learn this is not true....metastasis just means cancer that has spread.

I don't start to shake or sweat, I don't feel lightheaded. I just go to my desk, sit down and try to make sense of what I've just read. Then I do something worse, something I swore I wouldn't do anymore. I go to webMD.com and look up alveolar cell carcinoma. The results of my search add up to a horror show. I am certain now that I've just learned I'm about to die, probably having pieces of my lung removed surgically in the process.

I go to the bathroom, close the door behind me, and try to sit calmly without panicking. I feel as though I need to go somewhere, or under something, to try to somehow shield myself, but I quickly see that this is as good as it gets, in the bathroom, on the bathtub edge, with the door closed. Will Luke grow up without a father? How will I tell my own father, and mother, and family, and wife and friends, many of whom have never even seen me smoke a cigarette (one thing I glean at the web MD horror show is that this cancer is virtually always caused by smoking).

At the end of the first page of the radiology report under "IMPRESSION" the crux of the bad news is reiterated IN CAPITAL LETTERS. I turn to page two and it says simply "thank you for this referral."

Again, I want to tell no one and everyone. I decide to go out and buy the CD labels I promised Luke I'd apply to the kid's music CD I made for him last week, but first I stop off at my house to change my sweater. I have a lunch date at one o'clock, which I decide to keep, thinking distraction will do me well.

When I sit down on my bed at home it hits me. I feel a sorrow deeper inside me than I've ever felt and I start to weep. This is what it must feel like when you've killed someone and you first sense the irreversibility of what you've done. Or your first night in jail, when they close the door to your cell behind you. Time is now my master and it will give me as much or as little of itself as it pleases. Each wail seems to rise through a wide tunnel in my throat, then push itself out through my mouth.

My cell phone rings. It's a recent acquaintance, which forces me to go back to acting like everything's fine. A lucky break to get out from that dark mood. Later I call Steven and tell him. I read the radiologist's report over the phone. I can hear him going into shock, until he sort of raises his voice and says: "let's get one thing straight… no making any assumptions."

He explains that the reason a radiologist's report reads like a death sentence is that their job is to raise any and all possibilities so that they don't get sued. Patients aren't supposed to read the report, doctors are.

Four hours later, I walk into the office of Dr. Stuart Garay, pulmonary specialist. I start to tell him what I know and he interrupts me to say: " Steven Druckman called and said you're his best friend. He takes care of my kid," which is Jewish doctor-speak for "welcome to the *Mishpacha* (family)." His office and desk are so cluttered that if cleanliness were a measure of competence, he would now officially be a quack. Fortunately I see a sign on one shelf that reads: "I'm too busy to be neat," so at least he knows how insane he is.

He walks me through the CAT scan pictures, saying that normally the lungs look black with white streaks but as the photos head toward the bottom of my body (they are cross-sections taken at five millimeter intervals) there is a whiter mass which begins to be visible. The mass could be a tumor or a cyst or just a minor episode of pneumonia "resolving itself." I'd had a persistent cough for a month back in the fall that might explain the pneumonia idea. As he goes to slap up another sheet of scans on his light box, his fingers get all fumbly and the scan falls into a narrow slit between his desk and the wall, or more specifically, into the one spot where we will surely never see it again. Garay is genuinely embarrassed as we try in vain to get the huge desk with its piles and piles of papers and books to budge from the wall. "This is so embarrassing and that's the one photo we really need," he says. He calls maintenance in the building. As we sit and wait for five minutes while various colleagues of his stop in to see our absurd dilemma, I can't stop laughing, and I tease Garay about having bought the expensive desk made of the fancy heavy wood.

Eventually a Polish guy, who could probably lift the Space Shuttle if called upon, shows up and moves the desk. Garay says "Yeah...and us two Jewish weaklings couldn't move it an inch."

He goes back to his somber spiel and tells me: "You're a film maker. So don't play this out till the end of the film. Let's just take it one step at a time."

Play this out till the end of the film? I'm already thinking about the sequel, only guess what? There is no sequel. For the past half-hour I've been hearing the music from *Love Story* in my head, and thinking of how Ryan O'Neal starts the movie saying: "What can you say about a twenty-five-year-old girl who died?" One thing you can say is this: "She will not be in the sequel."

Garay is going to show my pictures to Doctor Schlossberg at New York University (NYU) Medical Center, who will eventually do a thin needle biopsy on my lung while Faust will handle the liver. We agree to talk the next morning after Schlossberg's seen my case.

The next day I go to NYU and have another identical CAT scan done by Faust's guy. This time Faust has asked them to inject me with a type of dye that helps provide contrast to the pictures. The technician tells me I may feel a warm sensation in my body, and a metallic taste underneath my tongue. He is a master of understatement. Within seconds, my blood feels like it is boiling, and I can feel adrenaline rushing through my whole body. There are no flames anywhere, yet I'm convinced that I'm on fire. The metallic taste under my tongue (probably like chewing Reynolds Wrap) only heightens my confusion.

My body temperature stabilizes at about a thousand degrees as I pass through the donut of the machine. Snap, snap, snap. The whole test is over in a couple of minutes. They send me home and tell me to be sure to drink a lot of water in the next twenty-four hours to flush the dye out from my system. I say: "Thank you," because I can't say what I'm thinking, which is: "Thanks for the miserable experience."

At some point I've got to tell my parents what's going on. Since I too am a parent, I know that they will be devastated no matter what I say. So I go through several scenarios in my head as to when would be a good time. I'll wait for the results of the new CAT scan. I'll wait until after my biopsy. I'll wait until I have a sure diagnosis. I call Steven to ask his opinion and he says: "Look man. Sooner or later you're going to have to tell them. At least if you tell them now, you won't have to obsess anymore about when to tell them."

He's right. I decide to call my mother first. She's less of a worrier than my father. Plus my father lives in town and I want to tell him in person.

"Mom. I've been back and forth to a bunch of doctors this week because I had a check-up and a bunch of tests and they now think I've got something on my lungs and my liver."

I listen for signs of breathing on the other end of the line. Just then my call-waiting indicator goes off and I say: " Mom I need you to hold because this could be my doctor." I hit the flash button and it's Faust on the other line. "Michael I have some potentially good news," he says, "I've got the results of the CAT scan and the radiologist now feels that the thing we saw on your liver is actually on your kidney. It's probably just a cyst, although quite a big one, but they are extremely common and non-threatening and we don't even treat them." He says to be sure I'll need to have a sonogram done. He has a guy he likes to use, and he'll make the appointment for me. I beg off the phone with Faust, then get back on with my mother. This is incredibly good news.

"Mom, that was my doctor. He said now they think I probably don't have anything on my liver which is, like, fantastic news." I can't believe how quickly my fortunes have just changed. My mother, meanwhile, has probably felt every possible human emotion in the span of about 45 seconds. She is badly shaken, but at least things seem to have taken a turn for the better. That night I go up to my father's house and break the news to him. He too tries to take comfort in the positive news about my liver.

On Monday I go to a Doctor Subramayan's office for my sonogram. Inside, it's basically me and about 15 pregnant women.

They lay me down on a table and a female technician rubs the metallic head of the sonogram over and around my abdomen. She points me to a monitor and says: "You see this? That's your liver. There's nothing there. Now look at this." She moves the gizmo down lower and to the right. "That's your kidney. That big thing that looks like a hole is just a cyst. It's nothing to worry about." I say: "Are you sure?" and she says, "Yes. I'm completely sure." I say: "Am I pregnant?" and she says, "No, you're definitely not pregnant."

No matter how bad my lung lesion plays out, this means I probably don't have metastasized cancer. I may have to pass through Hell to get to the other side, but I'll probably live.

Pulp Fiction

Today is my needle biopsy. I'm nervous, though not in a shaky, hard way. I just feel like I'm wearing a hat, even though I'm not.

The biopsy happens in the radiology section of NYU hospital. My friend Michael Kasino comes with me. As you enter and get your first look at some of the patients, you realize you're in the business end of the hospital – the heavyweight division. I actually see someone who looks either dead or five minutes from it, a woman on a gurney with a body complexion gone yellow. I fill out some brief forms. They seem to get briefer the worse your condition becomes, as if questions about the "why" of your presence are hopelessly redundant.

Schlossberg greets me with a Popeye-like handshake. Overstrong, reassuring, not the kind of grip to slip up during a procedure, though unfortunately not the kind of supple, piano-player-type hands that would imply a delicate precision for the upcoming biopsy. Hands that could drive a stake into you as efficiently as a needle.

He has a clipboard with a tome-like consent form. He tells me the risk of the biopsy is that my lung will collapse, and would I please sign right here. I don't bother to read the consent form (Fuck, the guy just said my lung might collapse, what further nightmare could be in the consent form?). I just sign it and ask him "what's your batting average?" He says only eight percent of people suffer a collapse, and only one percent of that eight percent need treatment for it.

I slip into a standard-issue gown that could easily be mistaken for your Aunt Trudy's tablecloth and head to registration. Even though there are only two people ahead of me, it takes a full thirty minutes to officially sign in (my sign-in takes five minutes, the wait to sign-in takes twenty five). Moments later Steven shows up. He's between his Brooklyn and Manhattan offices and has stopped by to see me. He brings word that they're looking for me back in Biopsyland and says: "Schlossberg thinks you've escaped."

At last, I'm led into my CAT scan room, sat down on the gurney and prepped. A doctor Gleason – young, good-looking – shaves a bit of my chest hair and tells me that a collapsed lung is what is called a pneumothorax and only one in ten people get it. I tell him that a pneumothorax sounds like a Dr. Seuss character and I think to myself that a few minutes ago, only one in twelve and a half people got one. My odds just got worse.

I get three quick injections of local anesthesia. The first one goes across my chest and burns a bit. The next one is vertical, and Dr. Gleason says: "Now a deeper burning." Suddenly the first burn is gone because the second one is worse. Then a third injection, a bit deeper, and Gleason says: "Even deeper burning." "Ow!" I add to the conversation. I flash on my father, who used to say to us when we'd complain of, say, a shoulder ache, "Want me to hit you on the head so your shoulder stops hurting?"

I'm sent under the scan donut a couple of quick times. Much to my dismay, they have no trouble finding my lesion. A recurring theme seems to be emerging in my ordeal, namely that the good news is always that they've discovered the bad news. Incredibly, I am really lucky that whatever I have has been found at all. There is some abnormal tissue on my right lung (and NOT on my liver, I keep reminding myself) and some routine chest X-ray led to something totally unrelated and practically non-existent (oh what I'd give for an old granuloma right now!) and that in turn led to the discovery of my lesion. But it's hard to feel lucky now, in this moment, when the long run is so far away from the short run, and Novocain pinpricks are jabbing into my chest.

My instructions are to stay still, then when commanded to "breathe in, breathe out, stop breathing." Six or so snapshots later, Gleason draws a line to a point on my chest with some sort of body crayon, then starts to unpack the needle.

Ah, nomenclature! Oh, great subjectivity of language and expression! There is a skyscraper in Seattle called the Space Needle. There is your standard sewing needle for a fallen off button. And somewhere in between there is your thin biopsy needle. See how thin it is, so acupuncture-like in its girthlessness? So lacking in profile view. My quandary is that I forgot to inquire about the rest of its dimensions. My needle is so long, it looks like it's supposed to biopsy the person lying under me, only there isn't anyone lying under me.

Gleason inserts it into my chest a few centimeters at a time. The real discomfort starts as it passes through my pleura, which is the lining of my lungs. My breathing automatically becomes shallow because it hurts to suck in too much air. I'm quickly rushed under the CAT scan and photographed. Gleason then attaches a syringe head to the top of the needle and sucks up tissue, swishing the needle around furiously as he does so.

He and the "team" are off for a few minutes to look at the specimen under the microscope. Someone stays behind to take another scan, which reveals that Dr. Seuss has just set up shop in my lung. I have a pneumothorax. It's a partial collapse, I'm told, nothing to worry about (compared to what, I can only wonder). Since it's now Schlossberg who's addressing me, I get the distinct feeling that Gleason kind of blew it. Schlossberg says: "We're gonna do one more pass and then we're done." "Another scan?" I meekly hope. "No, with the needle," says Schloss.

He steps to my right and jabs the needle in with his iron mitts and the cool nonchalance of a guy who never misses. I can practically see surrender in the eyes of my abnormal tissue. I barely make out my reflection in the glass covering the laser of the CT machine and I remember Steven telling me that my biopsy was going to be "like Pulp Fiction, that scene where Uma Thurman's overdosed on smack and they jab that huge needle of adrenaline into her chest. Exactly like that." I had assumed he was joking.

I take my umpteenth trip into the donut. Breathing is becoming harder and harder and it hurts like hell. The needle is in me like an unevictable tenant. Yet I think to myself: "Hey man, this sucks but I'm all right. It's bad but I'm all right." Schloss makes a direct hit on his first try. He does the syringe swish, yanks the whole thing out, and I'm done. He probably pretends to use the CAT scan as a guide just so Gleason and the others won't feel too inferior. Long live the Biopsy King. I'm wheeled out on a gurney and left to lie for a couple of hours on my stomach. They tell me not to move, and I stupidly try not to move *at all* which works if you're one of those Indian guys who spends his life doing yoga, but in my case just leads to cramping in my neck and back. A couple of chest X-rays later, Schloss says my lung's properly reinflated and he sends me home.

For a couple of days my right lung feels like a poorly hung coat. So far there's no diagnosis. Garay calls me with the news/no news, but the second time I press him. He's leaning toward a lymphoma diagnosis. It's almost certainly not benign. It might still be a carcinoma, which he says is what I'd call "cancer." As the conversation stretches on, I can palpably feel my happy options run out like a closing tap. I have what we have been euphemistically referring to as "the bad stuff." I just don't know how bad. Later on Steven tries the blunt approach, telling me not to wait till Tuesday, but rather to accept that I've got something in my lung and that it needs treatment. As far as I know, the big three of treatment are surgery, chemotherapy, and radiation. I decide to be courageous and ask what chemo and radiation really are. Chemo is an intravenous drug, highly toxic, which makes you nauseous and gives you basically the worst flu of your life. Your hair falls out and you lose your appetite, to name just a couple of its many awful side effects. Radiation can burn your skin, plus it can cause other cancers itself. Surgery (I finally dare to ask) is nasty, and painful once it's over. While not as dramatic as the crack of the ribcage done during heart bypasses, the ribcage is somehow penetrated and the operation proceeds.

What does all this mean? It appears the random test of a few weeks ago has now led me into a brotherhood of gloom and misery. Or it means I'm about to live the most meaningful and instructive period of my life. The bag comes mixed, I'm finding, and I feel an almost perverse curiosity about the depths of despair coupled with constant nervousness over each moment to come. There's already a psychological battle going on inside me between the introspective and the "outrospective", i.e. I'm scared but I'm simultaneously watching myself being afraid and questioning it. Am I afraid to die or am I afraid to have to confront mortality and to accept that maybe I'm not going to get hit by a bus, or have an aneurysm suddenly explode in my brain, or perish by some other instant means? I remember reading once in Jung something to the effect that man is a creature that lives in terror of self-knowledge. Steven tells me of essays he's read by terminal cancer patients and the one abiding principle of their memoirs is that none of them would ever have wanted to have gone through life without the experience of cancer. Part of me responds to that by thinking: "I guess cancer does warp your brain." I suppose I might better understand this particular idea of an invaluable experience were it coming from a survivor of cancer. But from terminal patients?

Meanwhile back on the Ranch of My Terror, I keep flashing on something Garay repeated to me: "What you have is probably treatable." Steven says he means "curable", in other words, totally possible to eliminate. But the more I think back on our talk, the more I sense something different in his tone of voice. To me, Garay's speech had virtually none of the characteristics of reassurance to it. Steven's trying to reassure me, Garay seemed to be saying something else.

Interpretation is becoming an awful burden. I try to listen closely and stifle the voices in me which just go on and on about "you're dead, you're not, you'll live, you won't, it'll hurt, it won't," and so on. Meantime I come up with these good reasons to have cancer:

1. You don't need to worry about your cholesterol for a while.

2. You can be sitting and thinking about something as trivial as an upcoming basketball game you want to watch, and people assume you're bravely and deeply reflecting on mortality and life's grand questions.

3. You might be offered sex by some sympathetic soul.

I start to imagine an unscrupulous movie character that tries to hustle up whatever he wants by pleading: "Please. I just found out I have cancer." Everything from a free plane ticket to a hand job from the passenger next to him, as in: "I'm really sorry even to ask for this, but I just found out I have cancer."

On Friday Garay said that he was leaning towards a diagnosis of lymphoma, though the final lab results wouldn't be ready until Tuesday. Steven chose to force me to face the facts. The weekend was hellish mostly because I had to keep facing my illness without knowing if it was carcinoma of the alveolar cells (i.e. a smoking related cancer) or lymphoma, or whatever else they have on the new menu at Chez Cancer. Now I know for sure – I have lymphoma. I'm relieved that this is totally unrelated to smoking – a clear conscience can go a long way toward sustaining the fighting spirit I'll need to muster.

Bad To The Bone

Day Two of me officially walking the planet with my three centimeter friend. Today begins the next series of tests to determine if the lymphoma is present anywhere else in my lymphatic system.

This morning on the radio I hear: "Police say a woman who was pushed out her window and fell twenty-one floors was not killed by her boyfriend pushing her. She was already dead after being stabbed fifty-one times by her boyfriend." I double-check the story in the *New York Times* and it turns out to be a grandson and grandmother. There's also an item about a twenty-five-year-old kid out in Central Park with his girlfriend. Three guys walk up, take his money and then as an afterthought, the fifteen-year-old among them puts a bullet in the guy's head and kills him. I read into this a simple message: I'm not that dead guy. I'm still alive, even though my life changed just as suddenly, mine on the end of a telephone, his from a gun connected to some kind of fucked-up childhood.

My therapist thinks I should talk to my son. Steven and my wife Layla think not. The real trouble is I don't feel comfortable telling my friends or family about the tumor because I don't want them leaving well-intentioned but sorrowful messages on my answering machine at home. I've got the best friends you could ever hope for in your life, and even if they are discreet, they'll still call, which means I'll have hours of phone time or heaps of messages to return. And obviously, this is not the kind of news you deliver in an e-mail message. I can just imagine that idiotic AOL voice going: "You've got cancer!"

My brother-in-law has already e-mailed me some supposedly "helpful info" on lymphoma but until you're the actual patient it's not possible to know how scary "helpful info" can be, because it just gives you facts without any real perspective. Still I can't resist. I open one of the e-mail attachments entitled simply "lymphoma." It says rather matter-of-factly: "Some lymphomas are indolent, which means the patient can live for many years without any treatment at all. Others are very aggressive, and among the most deadly cancers known."

Translated into patient-ese, it means, "You are about to die. Slowly perhaps, but surely." I assume this isn't the helpful part of the info, but then, how are you going to console me now that you've assured me of my imminent demise? My advice now to my friends and families is: inform yourselves, and then keep it to yourselves unless I ask for it. Meantime I'll ask my doctor instead of friggin' Google!

Dr. Garay has referred me to a hematologist/oncologist named Bruce Raphael. We go up to see him at his office at NYU. He doesn't much stand on formality – to say the least – he just sort of shakes my hand, then Layla's, sits us down and gives us the ABCs of lymphoma. I've got an accumulation of lymphocytes in my lung, he says. The big question is this: did they first accumulate here or were they sent from elsewhere? My fate rests almost entirely on this otherwise mundane question. Because I have no symptoms, and the testing that's been done on me so far shows no other presence of tumors, it appears unlikely that these bad boys are working for someone else. The rub is that the only way to know is through further testing. If this theory holds up, I'm looking at surgery (a.k.a. resection) and probably nothing else. Because lymphoma tends to recur I wouldn't get chemo until there were something new to try to kill or treat. Raphael says maybe he'd give me one chemo pill, sort of a Chemo Lite which wouldn't even cause my hair to fall out. He says if I were sixty he might not treat this at all, because I'd be more likely to die *with* it, than *of* it. So again this paradox arises, I feel great, I look great but I'm sicker than most people on the planet.

Raphael is reassuring so I pray he's right. I go into his treatment room, lie on my side, and go through a bone marrow sampling procedure. First a shot of Novocain in the hip, then two big needles (I carefully avoid looking at them) which go into my bone with the grace you'd expect of metal on bone, namely, lots of shoving which feels like grinding. This is considered a really agonizing procedure. The way to tell is that when you ask them to describe it, they always begin by telling you: "You'll live through it." For me it's an important moment psychologically. I've got to confront the issue of pain management and I'm a bit of a wuss in this regard. I mind needles, I mind discomfort, and I especially mind pain. Perhaps it's an outgrowth of my reluctance to use painkillers. I mean, I use them, sure, and there was one in particular called Talwin, a synthetic heroin I got when my wisdom teeth were extracted twenty years ago, whose prescription I gleefully finished long after the soreness was gone, but I believe in pain as a signal of recovery and thus a good regulator of activity. In short, pain tells you what you can and cannot do. But, pain in testing is just excruciating and serves no larger function outside of making you miserable.

I breathe like a madman, or rather like a woman giving birth, and it makes the discomfort manageable. By this I mean that I'm telling jokes instead of being unhappy. It helps enormously to have something to bear down onto, which for me is the table I'm lying on. I squeeze its edge with all my might.

When it's over two great things happen. First I am weirdly exhilarated and I discover a new confidence in myself. I've been saying all along that I'd get through this entire ordeal, now I begin to believe it. The second thing is that Dr. Raphael tells me that I could live a normal lifespan with this disease. The only news I've ever received of a comparable marvelousness was: "It's a boy." I'm ready to fight to live a normal lifespan. I suddenly envision all the milestones of Luke's life in my future, his first girlfriend, his first car, his college graduation.

I'm a warrior now. All it took was a glimmer of hope.

The General's Son

Because my parents are still living, Luke often says to me: "Dad, even though you're a Dad, you're still a kid." I have never been more aware of this in my life than I am presently.

I was born on May 27, 1960 at Beth-El Hospital, in the Flatbush section of Brooklyn, the son of first and second generation Americans whose parents in turn came from Ukraine, Poland, Romania, and Austria. Several of my grandparents and their siblings were draft dodgers. All of them were Jewish. Somehow this combination led to most of them becoming involved in the clothing business, which is to Judaism what law enforcement is to Irish Catholics, namely, the family business. Amongst ourselves we call it the *schmatta* business, as it's known in Yiddish; to non-Jews we call it the rag trade, and to impress people we use its more legitimate sounding name — the textile business. One grandfather was a tailor; the other was a menswear salesman. The tailor was poor, the salesman made a nice living. The tailor had a son, my father, who himself prospered in the retail garment business. The salesman had a daughter, my mother, who married the son of the tailor, and they in turn had two sons and a daughter before divorcing, one of those sons being me.

I grew up an army brat. Beginning in 1972, we moved to a new town every two years, though unlike most army families, we didn't move to places with names like Fort Bragg, or Fort Dix, or Fort Myers. We moved to fancy neighborhoods in New Jersey, and Los Angeles, and eventually San Francisco. My father had enlisted in the Jewish army, which is a pretty good description of what the retail clothing business is like. A lot of Jewish guys shouting at each other about strategy.

The difference is that in the Jewish army you don't learn how to cut your enemy's throat; you learn how to cut your overhead.

The closest our family ever got to the real Army was an encounter my grandfather Louis had during the Second World War. He flew from New York to Topeka, Kansas for a secret meeting with a guy in the Air Force. His plane landed in a cow pasture. My grandfather made a deal with his contact to buy a slew of used parachutes, which would then be reconfigured for use in the Jewish Army. Only instead of, say, thousands of Jewish paratroopers jumping out of aircraft behind enemy lines, my grandfather had a far more practical mission in mind. The parachutes were made of nylon, and nylon was nowhere to be found in America during the war. Back on 34th Street, my grandfather's company, Tanbro Fabrics, stripped the parachutes and made a mint selling real nylon underwear, and my grandfather returned home a hero. No ticker tape parade for him, of course, but I'm pretty sure he got a decent raise.

My father too signed up for a lifetime hitch in the Jewish Army, and each time we moved it was because of a new job he'd found which offered higher pay and more prestige. He eventually worked his way up to the presidency of a department store, which is roughly the equivalent of Four Star General, although he was eventually defeated in a coup d'etat (i.e. he got fired) and he moved on from retail into wholesale and manufacturing.

I was Bar Mitzvahed when I turned thirteen. I'd been brought up with what's called a conservative Jewish education, which means we followed a type of Judaism that conformed to certain realities of life in 20th century America, namely that Jews were still not well-liked, but they could find acceptance in American society if they'd lay off the beards, and the funny hats, and the kosher dietary laws, except for Passover which was more palatable, so to speak, because it was similar to Lent.

My parents never gave up hope that I would marry a Jewish girl. It wasn't forced upon me per se, I was just meant to understand that there'd be a hell of a fight if I decided to marry someone non-Jewish. When I first began dating, at age 16, it was with a girl who could properly be described as the consummate non-Jew (or *shiksa*, in Yiddish) – a platinum blond from a church-going family whose father was a colonel in the US Army. The *real* army. Her family smiled upon our relationship for nearly a year, until they found out about the non-stop sex we were having with each other, whereas my family was hip to the frolicking but likely saw this as a good chance for me to air out my sexual proclivities before someday meeting a nice Jewish girl I could eventually marry. One of my father's friends once remarked about the blond girl: "I know she's not Jewish, Mike, but she's got an incredible body." His point was quite clear and, in my opinion, representative of how the Jewish tribe looked upon my teenage romance. I was too young to marry – so I may as well get the temptation out of the way. Marriage could wait until I was finished wanting sex.

I used to believe in God. I think. I had this idea in my head that God would reward me with life if I behaved the way I was supposed to, or he would see to my sudden death if I did not. My first Hebrew school teacher, Mr. Arnold Kerns, used to keep a cardboard box full of individually wrapped candies on his desk. If we answered a question about Jewish history or ritual correctly, he would say in his terse voice: "Take one," and we would get to go up to the box and pull out our sugary prize. Looking back, I can see that Mr. Kerns was a deity of sorts. He spoke to us as if he'd been endowed with heavenly power, and he indeed had control over the thing that mattered most to a class full of six-year-olds –– candy.

The funny thing about your religious convictions is how quickly they race to the surface of your consciousness when something bad happens to you. Even though I'm now an atheist, I still know what it feels like to wish there were someone you could call upon when you find out you've got lymphoma. I don't mean a friend or a loved one – I mean some Being who might be able to exert some measure of control over a situation gone horribly wrong.

I won't lie to you – it's a really hollow feeling to be without that otherworldly Someone. Emotionally I can understand why people pray; I just don't get it intellectually. Yet there are some things in life that I have no intellectual answer for either. If you were to ask me how the miracle of childbirth happens, not the facts of fertilization, but the absolute miracle of the genesis of a human being, I don't think an intellectual, or scientific rationalization really explains much. It kind of reminds me of when I was a kid, and my parents would answer my questions about why I had to do certain things by saying: "Because I said so." Practically, this made sense; emotionally it was meaningless.

I have a confession to make. I also say: "Because I said so" to my son. I try to say it as sparingly as possible, but sometimes being a parent feels like a non-stop interrogation. Often I'm not even sure what crime my son is interrogating me about, although Henry Miller once wrote that all parents are guilty of the crime of bringing a child into this world in the first place.

I think that parenthood has finally given me a sense of a world larger than the confines of my mind and my body. I often look at Luke and think that he is at once a window to the future and a mirror of the past. He is constantly taking the elements of the world he sees and rearranging them into a puzzle that makes sense to him. All he really knows, at age six, is possibility. If he has any fear of death, it is probably just a fear of disappointing his parents. Death to him is just somewhere you go when you're one hundred years old (one hundred is *the* big number to a kid).

One thing I've learned about parenthood is this: it's very difficult, but for a reason I'd never expected. Before I became a father, I was worried about the burdens of having someone so dependent upon me. Human babies are the only creatures on earth that take years to become independent. They need to be fed, burped, changed, coddled, taken out, watched constantly, until at last they develop some modicum of independence, at which point they begin to need braces, and piano lessons. This is the stuff I was afraid of.

Yet once my son was born – probably within the first thirty seconds of his life – I realized that I'd been misled all along about parenthood. The hard part isn't having someone so dependent upon you. The hard part is *you* becoming so emotionally dependent upon *someone else*. There is no way to know in advance how profoundly a child can change you, or how truly precious they will turn out to be. And the more precious something is to you, the more powerful your fear of losing it becomes.

I feel as though I'm stuck between two fears: I'm afraid of losing, and of being lost. Like Luke says, even though I'm a Dad, I'm still a kid.

Get Me Rewrite

Here's a list of places you don't want to get cancer:

1. The brain

2. The throat

3. The testicles

4. The spinal column

5. The mouth

6. The colon

7. The pancreas

8. North Korea

The reason I make lists like this is to remind myself that things could always be worse, just as there's probably someone in Pyongyang waking up this morning saying: "Sure dictatorship sucks, but at least I don't have lymphoma."

This week the only testing I have is a PET (Positron Emission Tomography) scan up at Columbia Presbyterian Hospital – in an ultra modern wing still under construction. It goes like this: I'm injected with a radioactive dye, told to lie absolutely still and silent for fifty minutes as my body absorbs the dye, then I'm sent for another hour to lie just as still and quietly under a machine that looks like a boxier version of the CAT scan. I remember protesting nuclear power plants when I was in my twenties, and yet here I am willingly being injected – *into my veins, no less* – with nuclear waste, or rather, a radioactive isotope. So much for the grand ideals I held in college.

Michael Kasino comes with me again. Kasino's one of my best and oldest friends. The only friend I still have from college. He's smart, funny, and he's either come with me, or offered to come with me on every single medical appointment I've had so far. Really a true friend.

He also never shuts up. Believe me, I never shut up, so I know how to recognize it in others.

As I lay on the table, focused on stillness and inertia, he reads to me from the *Times* magazine section about a 15-year-old kid who made a mint hyping bullshit stocks on the Net. He reads me the gossip section on page 6 of the *New York Post,* which he loves but which bores me to death. I'm too afraid to tell him to shut up because any movement of my vocal chords, I've been instructed, could lead to a false positive in my test. I hold my tongue and try to give him a look that says: "Please shut the fuck up." That doesn't work, so I try a less polite: "Shut the fuck up" type of look. But it's useless.

The one truly great thing Kasino does is give me periodic updates on how much time I have left. I am dying to know, there's no clock in the room, and I've lost all track of time lying on this slow moving tray. He'll never know how much he helped me by doing something as simple as he did. I'm learning that it's good to bring someone with me for just this sort of inadvertent but critical help.

All I have left now is an endoscopy on Monday and my latest results and diagnosis on Wednesday. And of course the colonoscopy, the planning of which started this whole mess in motion. This has been my week of "mental remission," psyching myself up and feeling pretty good. Telling the last few friends I'm gonna tell.

I'm really scared these tests will show more evidence of lymphoma elsewhere, and so my wish becomes that I can at least start treatment from Stage One. From here on out it's gonna suck no matter what. There'll be differing opinions, less-than-concrete test results, and then weeks and weeks of whatever they dish out to the lymphatically-challenged.

Meanwhile, I spend a lot of time revising the daily story I tell myself about myself. I have to refer to it so often because I'm constantly asked how I am by everyone. The elements of the story are:

1. Who I think I am.

2. Who I hold responsible for my shortcomings and my pain.

3. How far ahead I am looking and how much hope I have invested in my future.

4. How far back I am looking and how much of my past I choose to carry with me.

My survival is all contained in my story. Do I wake up feeling that life is just a series of inevitable paroxysms like death or illness? Am I thinking that the cancer inside me may have already spread, and in any case, is known for its tendency to recur? As honest as everyone may be with me, are they saying to themselves and each other: "Michael may die," or "Michael won't be around that long," or "Michael is going to be horribly sick?"

Every morning I am editing my story, first for presentation to myself, then for the consumption of others. It's something we all do, everyday, but now I'm rewriting and editing so much more consciously. I honestly don't mind facing myself, I almost enjoy it sometimes, like when I feel hopeless and can still get myself to suck in some deep breaths and say: "Fuck it, I'm hopeless. Who isn't, except maybe a child?"

Learning To Love Snakes

"You've got MALT lymphoma," says Doctor Raphael, and I immediately envision a chocolate malted in a thick, fluted glass with a candy-striped straw. We are talking on the phone, which is when my mind tends to wander anyway. MALT stands for Mucosa Associated Lymphoid Tissue, which means it tends to show up in places lined with mucus. They're called Maltomas for short. When I'd first heard the MALT acronym thrown around a week ago, I began picturing malt liquor in my mind, specifically a green bottle of Mickey's Big Mouth beer, which I used to drink when I was a teenager and wanted to get drunk for cheap. The switch to the chocolate malted image comes as a surprise, although I've probably made some sort of association between milk and its propensity to produce mucus. I guess these are just my brain's feeble efforts to relate to a completely foreign concept.

The Positron Emission Tomography (PET) scan results are now in, and they show that the tumor is in my lung but I have nothing anywhere else (!). So Raphael's opinion is, let's operate and get the tumor out. He says there's an 80% chance it will show up again, and although mine is a chronic disease, it can be treated if it comes back. Who would ever imagine that the good news is that I'm going to have surgery? I am hugely relieved that there's no evidence of the cancer having spread. So I think I'm happy too, but I don't know if I trust any of my feelings anymore. I'm happy, I'm sad, I'm confident, I'm fearful. What I really am at this point – emotionally – is a three-year-old whose feelings change about as fast as you can say "ice cream." Give me ice cream and I will be happy. Otherwise, all bets are off.

Even so, I manage to act like an adult. I tell Raphael that although I believe him, I think it would be prudent to get a second opinion and he says to me, without hesitation: "Carol Portlock at Sloan-Kettering." I'm relieved because Carol Portlock is one of the oncologists who'd been suggested to me by a colleague of my brother's at his medical school (U.C. San Francisco) and also because I've been feeling a fair bit of trepidation about telling my doctor I want to second-guess him. Even though it is a standard practice in the world of medicine to get second, and even third opinions, doctors are as human as the rest of us, and no one likes being second-guessed.

Raphael also tells me that my bone marrow results are negative, and the CAT scan of my abdomen is normal. He says: "I can't promise you that a single undetectable molecule hasn't traveled somewhere else, but I couldn't test for it anyway even if it had."

Not so for Doctor Faust. I go to him for my endoscopy in the afternoon, exactly one week after my PET scan. I have been fasting all morning. Faust is great as always. I get some Demerol and Valium through a vein in my left hand, then a spray full of Lidocaine into my throat. I'm told to swallow and it tastes like....Lidocaine. Nothing you'd ever season food with.

My blood pressure starts a little high then settles down. I realize I'm not anxious about the procedure, but about what Faust may find. Maltomas tend to "present" (show up) in the Gastrointestinal tract. The odds are that my lung tumor isn't the primary spot, even though all the tests so far have been negative. Faust is also going to do some random biopsies of my stomach. He sedates me – a much lighter sedation than I'd anticipated, kind of like a good herbal tea and fire-in-the-hearth-type buzz – then shoves a metal tube down into my esophagus, a sensation probably not unlike fellating an AK-47. Through the metal tube he passes a thin cord with some type of gizmo at the end that can slice away and collect tissue samples. I feel a slight sensation of movement in my stomach as I lie on my left side. I emit a long monotonous burp from all the air he's pumped inside my gut and I drool copiously onto a drool towel. I'm a guy, so somehow I derive pleasure from all the burping. Go figure.

It's over in ten minutes. All he's found is a touch of gastritis – small, meaningless inflammation. The biopsies are sent off to the lab.

So here's what I'm looking at now. Raphael wants me to have surgery to get the tumor out. I'll see him on Saturday to get all the gory details. The tumor is beneath my rib cage so I'm guessing they're gonna have to crack some bones to get it, but I'm sticking to my policy of not wigging out until I'm sure of what to wig about. Tuesday I hope to go to Sloan-Kettering for a second opinion, but I'd be very surprised if they differed with Raphael. So far he's called a perfect game. My PET scan lit up at the site of the tumor and nowhere else, which is what he predicted.

Today I also begin prep for tomorrow's colonosocopy. Ah yes, that colonoscopy I'd worried over seemingly so long ago. Ironically, the exam that set this whole ordeal in motion will be my last one.

Prep can be summed up in one simple word - Void. I drink a full gallon of a kind of Drano for humans over a four hour period, set myself down in the bathroom for about enough time to read *War and Peace,* then for extra fun, I get to give myself an enema tomorrow morning. This for a guy who is still deeply traumatized from the time he visited his Nanna Rose in Florida, at age five, and received an enema as treatment for a mild bellyache. I'm certain that a little kiss on my tummy would have done the trick, but Nanna was one of the last great Jewish Mothers, who would give you an enema for any ailment from the neck down, and chicken soup for anything neck up.

I phone Garay to go over the options. Now that we think we know what's wrong with me, where should I get treatment? A second opinion is a prudent step particularly since I'm facing surgery. Carol Portlock is at Sloan-Kettering, which is to cancer treatment what UCLA once was to college basketball. In other words, the best. However, a quick call to her assistant reveals that she's booked for the next two weeks. Garay tells me: "You need to know the Pope if you're Catholic or God himself if you're Jewish to get an appointment up there."

Garay says he sent his relatives to Mort Coleman at New York Hospital, who has an international reputation, and who, according to an e-mail from my brother's friend at UCSF medical school, is an oncology fellow at Cornell. What would you do? Garay says he has one other person he wants to ask for an opinion and he'll get back to me as soon as he hears from him.

Professional recommendations are a tricky business as it is. I can't count the number of times I've been disappointed by people highly recommended to me. *Severely* disappointed. Like my plumber. Highly recommended. Disappeared in the middle of the job. Or my first car mechanic. The guy probably lives on a yacht thanks to all the money he bilked out of me. He was highly recommended by a good friend of mine. But doctors are different, right? They are recommended on the basis of their verifiable skills. Until one day they suddenly show up on the local news wearing handcuffs, accused of euthanasia, and speaking through their lawyers...

Then again, these are only my oncologists. Neither of them will perform the actual surgery on me, so this is just the first part of a two-part decision I need to make.

Fortunately, I cop a break. Two days later, Portlock's secretary calls and says there's an opening in a few days due to a cancellation, so I snag it. Five minutes later, Garay calls and says "his guy" says that between Mort Coleman and Portlock, I should go with Portlock, so I feel comfortable for now. Psychologically comfortable, that is. Physically I am otherwise engaged.

Colonoscopy prep sucks. The Drano-like beverage tastes like Gatorade that flunked quality control, but it's actually bearable until the last two cupfuls, in which the solution seems to have reconstituted itself and the horrible taste is now concentrated and unmerciful. But after 4 hours of slugging this gunk every 15 minutes, I'm not about to throw it up and have to start all over again.

For the next 3 hours, it all comes out, how shall I say it? Fountainously? Even the enema is not a big deal – a small, pre-packaged bottle. Just squeeze and wait ten minutes. It's hard to believe people do this voluntarily- they call it colonics. I call it deliberately lowering your quality of life. When the preparation is over, or rather, when I am certain that not one single atom of food or drink remains within the confines of my body, I get into bed and wait for sleep to overwhelm me. I like the idea that I am now as free from the tyranny of eating and drinking as I have ever been, and my body feels to me like a temple of purity, except for the one nasty spot in my lung.

The next afternoon I am back in Faust's office for the colonoscopy. The colonoscopy procedure is like having a metal snake slink up your ass (not that I have much experience to draw upon), but a combination of Valium and Demerol quickly turns me into an avid herpetologist. At one point Faust asks me how it's going and I say, slurring: "You can drive a truck up there for all I care. This Demerol's great!" I am not kidding. This very moment is now tied for nearness-to-nirvana with the moment that I woke up in a morphine stupor after having my wisdom teeth pulled twenty years ago. I am wasted, and loving it!

When it's over and the Demerol has worn off, Faust tells me that the stomach biopsies he took on his last trip through my gastro-intestinal tract are negative, and the colonoscopy now shows that I'm cool from the bottom down too. Since the PET scan is also negative, we know for sure that I've got a localized tumor in my lung. Period.

The Hot Iron

Leon Trotsky, the co-architect of the Russian Revolution, once said something to the effect that: "People respond to a tickle differently. But to a hot iron, alike!"

I get to Sloan- Kettering at a quarter to two, fifteen minutes early. I make like I'm going to walk in, then quickly invent some phony excuse to myself along the lines of "maybe I ought to eat something first." The truth is, this is when it hits me that I've got cancer. Finally. This is the hot iron. Right there at the door to the Memorial Sloan-Kettering Center for Cancer Research (MSKCC). All the testing, all the talk, all the denials....everything sort of evaporates when you stand at the entrance to this odd and awe-inspiring building. This place is here because of one disease only. It's a weird feeling of having finally arrived. I walk over to First Avenue into a few nearby food joints, but as I already know, I'm not hungry – I'm just freaked out. Eventually I muster my courage, head back east and walk in.

The first thing I see is a golden placard on the wall that says: "God's love and a courageous spirit will help to speed recovery." It is not comforting to me; rather, it is an ominous sign that there is trouble brewing in this building. And yet, it's a friendly place. All I can think is, the people around me also have cancer, save for the staff. Usually in a hospital you wonder who's sick and who's well. Not here.

Up on the fourth floor, in the lymphoma section, I'm examined by a Dr. Pan, a youngish Asian woman who's so thin she's practically invisible in profile. She reaches under my arms and says she's checking out my lymph nodes. There is no sign of swelling. A few minutes later, Doctor Portlock comes in, wearing a white lab coat. She has a longish, narrow face and a small mouth that doesn't move much when she talks. She introduces herself as Carol Portlock, which is the first time anyone has used his or her first name with me in place of "Doctor." She re-checks my lymph nodes, has me draw a couple of breaths while she listens with her stethoscope, then invites Layla and me to come into her office to talk.

She says she's seen the results of the various tests done on me and she concurs with Doctor Raphael's conclusion, namely that I ought to have the tumor resected.

Her opinion is that radiating this tumor would be dangerous because it's close to my pericardium (heart) and could inadvertently damage my heart. Plus radiation can itself cause other types of cancer. Portlock says I'm too young for those types of risks, and she blushes when I offer to kiss her for calling me young. I like her. Having my wife here with me is important because I'm doing what I call listening defensively. Speaking to your oncologist/hematologist, I'm finding, is like walking through a minefield. You never know if the next thing coming out of their mouth is going to be some new unforeseen horror or not. I listen as closely as I can, but I'm also simultaneously bracing myself mentally for whatever bullets she may be about to shoot. I'm sort of absorbing what I feel I can deal with so I need someone like Layla there who can corroborate the facts with me post-consult.

Portlock says she'll treat me if I want, and she's sure they have "a number of capable surgeons up to the task." I venture a query into the nature of the operation, and she gives me a few gruesome details. Incision among the ribs, tube sticking out of me for a few days, my lung collapsed, 4-5 days in the hospital and about a month till I'm back to normal. Just what I was afraid of.

The next day, I'm on the phone with Raphael who sums it up like this: "You're gonna feel like someone beat the shit out of you." But the upside is, this may be it...forever. Oddly, that's sort of my own personal history of getting the shit beat out of me, to this point. The last (and only) time was when a kid named Stan Olshefski clocked me in the jaw at a baseball field in New Jersey, because I argued with him about whether or not he was safe or out at home plate. I got on my bike and raced home in tears. I only wish I could do the same thing today.

Portlock says it'll be "a blip on the radar" of my life. Of course once they pull the tumor out and really examine it whole instead of just a few aspirated cells, things may change. Now that I know that radiation is like a six-week ordeal and chemo is something even harsher, I'm going to try to get psyched up about surgery. It's just not easy volunteering to get the shit beat out of you. I try to imagine what it would be like to go back to Stan Olshefski and ask him to hit me again.

To hear my father tell it, you'd think I just got nominated for an Oscar. I call him with the latest news and he's all: "Mike that's terrific. Aren't you thrilled?" Now I'm not saying I'm not glad I'm going to live, but terrific and thrilling just don't fit the occasion. Frightened but dealing is more my current vibe. Somehow I'm feeling indestructible, though, because if this isn't going to kill me, then what the hell will, right?

Friday I will meet Felix Heller, NYU thoracic surgeon. He and Steven go way back. Meantime, I'm having my brother dig up some names of Sloan slicers, and then I'll make the call. I also need to make up a will. Seriously.

My operation is supposed to cure me. Is there a risk that it will kill me? Probably a small risk. I wonder what will be the last thing I see before I go under and succumb to the anesthesia? Will it be a detail, like a light, or a nose of one of the doctors? Will I hear a strange sound like nothing I've ever heard before? Is there a signal before you go for good, like a warm sensation through your spine, or an inexplicable peaceful feeling behind your ears? Do you hear a discordant sound or sense a change in the color temperature of the light around you?

My therapist just told me that even though I don't believe in God, she does and she's praying for me. My Aunt Paula said she had her congregation speak my name in unison during their prayer for healing at synagogue last Friday night. A group of people unknown to me said: "Michael Solomon" to an invisible emptiness, hoping for me and hoping, I guess, that my salvation will confirm their belief in a controlling order to the things which frighten us most: death and disease, loss and suffering. While I can't join in their prayer to No One, I still feel good to be thought about, and invoked, and loved in some primordial way by a part of the human community.

Math And Meaning

This week I am mentally adjusting to surgery. I've been pretty calm, actually didn't psychologically "have" cancer for several hours the other day, meaning it was a surprise when I slipped back into "oh-that-annoying-monster" thought-mode. But I've been nagged by this doubt – am I maintaining a positive attitude or am I just in denial about the severity and prognosis of my illness? I'm asymptomatic and I don't think I even feel like a person with a serious illness, or disease. Or maybe the words are lacking in their ability to convince me. I'm viewing this as if it were a benign tumor – necessary to resect as Raphael says, but non-threatening. I guess the further irony, beyond that of being sick yet feeling terrific, is that my cancer is malignant and yet it hasn't spread anywhere (except perhaps a few molecules at a time to some undetectable place).

This then leads me to wonder about the wisdom of surgery. Is it my lymphatic system that has gone mad, or is it this one area of my lymphatic system and thus by removing it, the cause will be eradicated. If it were systemic, would the spread originate from the site of my current tumor? If not, what risk does my tumor pose? How large does it need to get before it causes me any problem? I'm not sure I understand the logic, although I do know that the resected tumor will allow for a more accurate diagnosis. But fuck – that's a lot of abuse just for a diagnosis. No one has quite put it this way, but I believe I'm having surgery in place of an open-chest biopsy. To what degree I do not know. I also don't know if an open-chest biopsy would really be much less invasive, but I'm going to ask.

I expend a lot of effort keeping my mind focused and ready, but a lot of that involves filtering information or avoiding it, a.k.a denial.

I find a lot of decent information at nhl.org- the non-Hodgkins lymphoma website I went to after accidentally visiting nhl.com- the official website of the National Hockey League.

I also learn a valuable lesson about survival statistics courtesy of an essay by Steven Jay Gould, the zoologist, and mesothelioma patient, concerning something called "median" survival rates. Median survival rates are expressed in years and percentages, like this (for example):

83% survival 5 years from diagnosis

50% survival 10 years from diagnosis

At first glance, you would think the odds of a person living another 5 years are good, but their odds of making it 10 years are only 50-50. While this is technically true, it is highly misleading.

For argument's sake, let's say that the median survival rate at 10 years is 50%. That means that half the people died at somewhere between 0-10 years from the time they were diagnosed. But the other half lived *at least* 10 years and often quite a bit more. Since I'm a person whose relative youth, strong constitution, early detection and lack of symptoms strongly favor my chances, I need to think of myself as having a far greater than 50-50 chance in such a hypothesis. For instance, say I'm one of six patients:

Patient #1 dies at ⟶ 1 year from diagnosis

Patient #2 dies at ⟶ 3 years from diagnosis

Patient #3 dies at ⟶ 5 years from diagnosis

Patient #4 dies at ⟶ 11 years from diagnosis

Patient #5 dies at ⟶ 33 years from diagnosis

Patient #6 dies at ⟶ 40 years from diagnosis

Here, half the patients (50%) are dead within 5 years, which means the median at 5 years is 50%. But the remaining three survivors lived for quite a bit longer, one of them a full 40 years more! So a 50% median survival rate doesn't mean therefore *I'll* be dead in 5 years or less. Gould's diagnosis of mesothelioma had a median survival of 8 months. He's now 20 years in and apparently doing great. Christ I hope so. As a cancer patient you get so invested in other patients' stories that you feel your destinies become intertwined, even with people you never meet but only hear about. It's like a real-life web page in which you're hyperlinked to everyone who has cancer. Deaths threaten you, triumphs inspire you.

Later I watch a webcast about nutrition and lymphoma. I quickly realize I don't have the patience to learn everything I need to know about nutrition. I just want someone to go: "Hey Solomon. Eat more sweet potatoes." Or whatever.

A few days later I have a dream. I am on my computer downloading something when a file called CHOP flashes onto my screen and I desperately fight to push "escape" to eliminate it. CHOP is a type of chemotherapy I read about.

Just in case I was able to consciously get myself into a positive and optimistic way of thinking, my subconscious wants me to know that it's taking notes about everything too.

Meet The Surgeons

Felix Heller's office has a design flaw. There's an entrance door that brings you into the waiting room. Another door leads to a corridor, along which are Felix's office, an examination room, and several other offices. But the waiting room has no receptionist's window. You have to sort of kneel on one of the chairs, stick your head through a makeshift window in the wall, crane your neck and look south. Luckily I run into Felix on my way down the main hall to the office. He kindly takes my by-now-voluminous set of films and reports and tells me he'll be with me in a second.

Steven and Felix go way back. I'm not sure if Felix mentored Steven when Steven was a young doctor, but it was something like that. Felix tells me Steven called him about me, which surprised him because Steven usually calls about pediatric cases, or "peeds" as Felix puts it.

First a word about Felix's secretary. Foxy. A red-haired beauty. Even in the world of cancer care you notice things like that. Now Felix. Kind. Paternal. Gray. Handsome. He gives me a quick physical exam (which by now I could do myself, if need be) then we go to his office and talk.

He explains he's going to give me a lobectomy. He'll make an incision about seven inches long between two of my ribs, use a spreader to pry them apart and give himself room to work, then remove the middle lobe of my lung. He says the middle lobe is the smallest part of the lung, responsible for only 3-4% of total lung volume, and it is the only part of the lung which, when removed, causes the other two lobes to expand into its space and thus compensate for lost volume.

He says he does several things to limit the post-op pain, so mostly I'll feel sore in front and back where the hinges of my ribs were stretched beyond normal. It's a fairly routine procedure (Garay later tells me he sends about one patient a week for a lobectomy) and in Felix's estimation, my chances of a recurrence in ten years will hover around zero percent. He will also remove the lymph nodes that act as conduits for homeless cancer cells.

The breathtaking ease with which he speaks of opening and ravaging my chest cavity is inversely proportional to the ease it provokes in me. Talking with a surgeon about surgery is like talking with a felon about crime – feeling becomes subordinate to technique. Mind you, Felix is a real gentleman – soft, comforting voice, non-trembling hands (you bet I'm checking!!), just the right mix of confidence and humility. At one point he says that while he's inside me, he'll check for any other occurrences on my lungs, and it's this expression: "while he's inside me," that makes me shudder.

I'm a thoracic virgin. My thorax has never been penetrated, save for a bit of foreplay during my thin-needle lung biopsy, but even that never felt like someone snooping around inside my chest cavity. Here I am now with a kind, soft-spoken gentleman giving me the details of a surgical fist fuck.

I ask Felix if this surgery will eliminate the base from which my cancer could spread and he says yes. Cancer spreads in three ways, either through direct contact with other tissue (i.e. a tumor makes its way into an adjacent area) or by traveling through the blood or by traveling through the lymphatic system. So this operation would definitely keep it from spreading. What I believe about lymphoma, which is what makes me skeptical about surgery, is that even though surgery will keep it from spreading, nothing can apparently stop it from re-appearing, fresh, at another time. I believe that surgery is the right treatment for me now; what's hard is not knowing the cause of my lymphoma in the first place.

Felix tells me there's a one-tenth of one percent risk of my dying during surgery. There's a one percent chance I'll develop an infection. I'll have three to four days in the hospital, and I'll wake up with a drainage tube sticking out of me, which they will remove at my bedside a few days later, then send me home for three to four weeks of ambulatory rest. Felix says I'll feel tired just from walking across the room, but pain-wise, a couple of Percocets a day or perhaps just steady Motrin should do it. The good news is there won't be any cracking or sawing through ribs as in cardiac surgery. No bathing me in ice to slow my heart down. However, I will be getting an epidural catheter, inserted into my spine, for pain control, so as long as I don't move I won't get paralyzed.

WHAT??

Fuck. There's just no getting off easy, is there? Once again, modern medicine proves to be miraculous, unless you're the vehicle for said miracle. Behold the wonders of the human anatomy, just hope you're not the window that everyone's looking through!

I tell Felix I'm still going to meet one other surgeon, and then I'll make up my mind and schedule a date. As I'm about to leave I remember one other question:

"Is my lung going to collapse?"

"We collapse the lung in order to operate on it," is his answer.

Gee thanks. I leave his office feeling much less frightened about the operation, though I obsess about the epidural a bit on my way home. My wife tells me she's had four epidurals – one during childbirth, and three more in a failed attempt to restart the healing process in her ailing knee. I guess I'll just endeavor to stay still when my time comes.

A few nights later I have a nightmare about Valerie Rusch (pronounced ROOSH), the surgeon from Sloan-Kettering I'm scheduled to see later in the week. In my dream, I'm at Memorial, as Sloan-Kettering is called (MSKCC for now on – CC stands for cancer care). A black doctor is talking to me and several other white doctors are crowded around, all of them obscuring Valerie Rusch. They're talking to me, but I can't see Rusch, until finally the crowd sort of separates and I see her. She is unusually young looking, maybe late twenties, with blond hair in a permed seventies style, and blue eyes. She looks like a girl who'd pass for pretty in, say, Dayton, Ohio. Valerie tells me in the dream that she has some sort of nasal condition so she can't treat me (which certainly refers to my now chronic stuffy nose that's been worrying me, or rather, that seems to me like a symptom of my illness because it too is mucus related), and also, says Dream Figure Rusch, she can't examine me because I've forgotten to bring my X-rays and CAT scans to the appointment. I can't believe I've overlooked such an important thing, and I am panicked that I have done something irreversible.

Then, thankfully, I wake up.

My therapist thinks I'm nervous about the surgery, and that maybe I'm nervous about having a woman operate on me. My wife is all in favor of a woman surgeon and oncologist because she says women pay more attention to the details.

It reminds me of the old riddle about the boy and his father who are driving in a rainstorm. Their car swerves and hits a tree. Two ambulances show up, and take the boy and his father each to separate hospitals. The father goes under the knife and recovers. But at the boy's hospital, the doctor who walks in to the operating room refuses to perform the operation. The doctor says simply: "I can't operate on that boy, because that boy is my son." So how is this possible? (answer: the doctor is the boy's mother)

I call Garay who says about Rusch: "She's excellent."

The day I actually go to see Dr. Rusch (thanks to a last minute cancellation) I take Layla and myself to the wrong facility; namely, Portlock's office up on 67th Street. Rusch is in the Rockefeller Pavilion on 53rd and Lex. It's probably ridiculous, but it feels like these sorts of small miscues have a tremendously large impact, especially when you're living with the feeling that anything.... absolutely anything...is possible from one minute to the next. We grab a cab, race down to 53rd and Lex (I envision a headline: "Lymphoma patient killed in auto accident on way to doctor") and arrive five minutes late.

American Airlines has a business class lounge at most major airports called the Admiral's Club. It is nearly identical to the office of Dr. Valerie Rusch, except that instead of laying over in Frankfurt, say, you're either hanging out waiting to enter the Chemotherapy Suite or to be examined by one of the thoracic surgeons. The wood furniture is modern Italian, a TV set plays CNN in one corner, computer terminals offer a chance to peruse cancer info on DVD, and an automatic mocha/cappuccino machine stands guard over cups and saucers and mini-bags of pretzels. And so on. The receptionists sit around a semi-circular open architecture set of tables and attend to patients like travel agents taking holiday reservations. They're all dressed in matching dark blue gowns like the ones the traders wear on the floor of the New York Stock Exchange. The announcement of an arriving flight would not seem in the least bit out of place here. Instead patient's names are announced, the way pages in snazzy hotel lobbies used to do it back in the Twenties, except that they don't ring a little bell when they call your name.

"Mr. Solomon?" "Mrs. Dobrynin?"

From the mix of foreign tongues you hear, it's evident that many people have come here from the four corners of the earth.

Layla looks around like a queen returned to her palace and says: "How civilized." She's right. The funny thing is, the most important decision in my life since where I wanted to attend college now seems to hinge upon the availability of hot espresso. Luckily, the application of frivolous criteria to a monumental choice is really nothing new to me. My decision to forego the University of California at Berkeley and instead attend UC Santa Barbara was made when, on a chance visit to the latter campus, the parking attendant emerged from her booth in a sexy bikini and a body from beach heaven. I applied for a transfer immediately. All in all, it was the right choice, even though I ended up having far, far less sex than I'd hoped for in college. I firmly believe that world leaders, on the basis of whether or not they got laid the previous night, make many, if not most fate-of-the-human-race decisions. Hell, it's a known fact. Why should I be any different when it comes to coffee and pretzels?

The truth is: such comfort is no accident. The MSKCC folks aren't being ostentatious. They're showing off that they know that coffee and pretzels *matter*. Comfort is important, because it's reassuring, and people with cancer are adrift no matter how strong they are. Cancer pulls the rug out from under you – whether or not you fall won't put the rug back in place for you. Things like coffee and pretzels give you traction on an otherwise slippery slope.

Inside Rusch's examination room, I'm given yet another gown to slip into, only this gown seems for a change like it wasn't manufactured by prison labor in China. The fabric is on the thick side, the color a respectable navy blue, and the belt of the robe even goes once around the back and ties in front like – dare I say –a robe! Suddenly I am not just Michael Solomon with lymphoma, I'm Hugh Hefner with a removable tumor.

A cocoa-complected nurse named Carolyn Sadler asks me the first round of questions. I retell my lame joke about how the only other member of my family having medical problems is my brother, who's struggling to get through medical school. I've told that joke to four different doctors and nurses now, and it gets worse with each new telling.

Next a youngish doctor named Charles Gibson comes in and examines me with his stethoscope. He looks to be in his early thirties, and I imagine not unlike how my brother will wind up. He speaks to me in a sort of doctor Haiku:

"Deep Breath."

"Again."

"Again."

"Good. Thank You."

At last Dr. Valerie Rusch walks in. She's younger than I expected though older than the woman in my dream. My guess is that she's somewhere in the thirty-seven to forty-two-year-old range. Not unattractive though not my type (Thank God! I've got enough problems.). She tells me she's of Swiss descent, which makes me think of clockwork and cleanliness and precision, although I know this is just wishful thinking. For all I know, she could have an uncle guilty of war-crimes hiding out in the Alps. Maybe I'll just focus on something neutral, like chocolate.

She says to me more than once: "We don't know exactly what you have. Could be an early stage lung cancer, though so far, it's consistent with lymphoma." She's going to try to resect my tumor and middle lobe using a thoracoscopy, which is a procedure involving a video-assisted device not unlike an arthroscope. She'll make two small incisions, each about an inch and a half long, one in front, one in back, and a third tinier incision on my side. One hole is for the camera, one is for her cutting tool…I don't remember what the third one's for but I know they don't need to use a clapper slate like we use in film so who knows…

If it works, I'll recover in no time. If not – and she expects it will not – she'll connect the front and back incisions, spread open my ribs, and pull it out the usual way. That's called a thoracotomy, which is basically the same as a lobectomy.

She says about five days in the hospital with a drainage tube sticking out of me, followed by a month or so to get back to normal. She's off to Paris next week, and I want to wait till after Luke's birthday, so we schedule April 5th for the main event. She pulls out her immaculate calendar and writes me into her schedule. I don't bother to tell her that I'm considering another surgeon, because as of this moment, I no longer am. Even though there's only a slim chance of the less invasive procedure succeeding, I don't feel I have anything to lose by letting her try it. Plus I've been hearing from my people on the grapevine – my brother's instructors at UCSF, and Doctor Garay here in New York – that Valerie Rusch has a reputation for brilliance.

Meantime, I am still the healthiest unhealthy guy I know. It's not an easy paradox to reconcile, especially when everyone is making such a point of telling me how "great" I look, and I keep telling them how "great" I feel. With all this good looking and great feeling going on, you'd think we were at a cocktail party in Hollywood. Or a funeral in Hollywood, for that matter.

No Quarter

It's a relief to finally have a date but -– hmm, seems like there's always a "but" – now it's time to face the risks of surgery. Like every other aspect of my condition, surgery gets far more threatening as it approaches, not just in the temporal sense, i.e. my surgery is only "x" days away, but more so in the microcosmic view of what it entails. The devil is in the details, as they say.

Surgery is safe. The vast majority of people don't die from it. Its pain is manageable. Drugs exist to blunt pain extraordinarily well. Surgery is effective. It can even be curative. Unfortunately, it's essentially irreversible. You can't reinsert part of your lung and more importantly, you can't undo the trauma your body and mind undergo. So what happens to someone like me when he buys the non-refundable ticket to the show?

To begin with, I have to deal with scary articles in the *New York Times* that feel like they've been written with me in mind. One headline screams: "**HEY MICHAEL!! FDA RECALLS RAPLON!!**" Raplon is a drug given along with general anesthesia to make it easier for surgeons to insert breathing tubes. Insertion of a breathing tube will be one of the opening gambits in my operation. The problem with Raplon, they've discovered, is that it causes far more severe bronchospasms than testing had revealed, and several people have now died because their airways constricted until they were totally closed. Doctors described their attempts to save these patients as "trying to ventilate cement" or "a brick wall." Call me paranoid, but honestly, I know none of those dead people went into surgery thinking they could suffer such a reaction, much less die from it. I'll be calling my doctor Monday morning just to be sure Raplon isn't still on the menu for me, although it's not very reassuring to think that Raplon was being used in the first place (I learn from the *Times* article) because it had fewer and less severe side effects than anything else!

Fuck! Have I said that before? Fuck!

I'm becoming Evel Knievel. I'm about to do something very dangerous and I'm likely to survive it, even though my vehicle, a.k.a. my body, will definitely be involved in a fiery wreck. Firefighters will be standing by. Gee, that's comforting. That's exactly what's so scary – the human element. Another article in the paper says between 44,000 and 58,000 people a year in the U.S. die from medical error.

WHAT?????

Yeah, don't worry Mike. You'll be fine. You're in great hands. And so on. Which reminds me, I still need to write up a will.

I go for pulmonary function testing at Garay's office. The idea is to set a benchmark against which I can check my breathing after my operation. My technician is a sweet-faced Ethiopian guy with an unpronounceable (and impossible to memorize) name. He was a medical student in Ethiopia, showed promise, was shipped off to Russia (Ethiopia's then-ally) for further studies, and wound up here in New York six years ago as a P.F.T. – pulmonary function technician. Garay says he's excellent and it's true – no pain at all when he extracts the bluish, oxygen-rich arterial blood from my wrist, despite the overabundance of nearby nerve endings which normally makes blood-gas testing like this excruciating.

We somehow get onto talking about the wireless world, and he tells me he'd like nothing more than to be able to monitor his car and his house, twenty four hours a day, on his P.D.A. He's totally serious. He's been traumatized by city life, and he says he's had his car broken into.

The PFT says he'd like to monitor his as-yet-unborn children like this too. Now I'm thinking: "This guy is a little weird." Is he – are we – so frightened for our kids in this day and age, or is technology just making it easier for us to avoid confronting, and overcoming, our fears? This is part of what I am experiencing. I don't want to place too much faith in technology.

I think generally it's really tough for me to feel "lucky" because I'm scheduled to go through a huge ordeal to rid me of something that doesn't bother me at all. Various experts and the tests they administer assure me they're only saving me (and even then, just hopefully) from an even worse ordeal.

I sit in a capsule not unlike something NASA might design, a plastic bubble, shaped like a gondola ski lift, within which a confluence of plastic tubes juts out in all directions from a console. A cylindrical mouthpiece in turn anchors the console. I get the impression I'm going to test-drive this thing, only with my mouth. I follow the PFT's instructions to breathe deep, push out, hold it, breathe deeper, and pant as I watch a computer screen graph trace my pulmonary efforts in rising and falling arcs. Later I'm made to breathe asthma medicine for seven minutes in order to assure my airways are at maximum functionality.

I'm pleased to learn that my lungs, except for the pesky tumor, are in good shape, which means I've thus far dodged the ill effects of having smoked cigarettes for 20 years. Once again, other than cancer, I'm in excellent health!

One week later, I go back to the Admiral's Club for my pre-admission screening. A nurse takes blood, another takes urine, and a doctor discusses anesthesia with me (no mention of Raplon). I'm given something called an incentive spirometer, which is not entirely unlike a bong without any water, and which operates on a similar principle.

In order to keep fluid from building up in the lungs after surgery, I'm supposed to give my lungs a workout by sucking air in through my spirometer at a constant rate. I put the mouthpiece in, and then try to breathe in deeply and steadily. A tiny yellowish button is drawn up through the spirometer by the force of the air I breathe in (the air is invisible…. were this a bong, we would *see* the pot smoke traveling from the bowl into the main chamber of the bong and on upwards), until it reaches a level that's been indicated with, of all things, a smiley face icon. I'll need to take ten hits…I mean breaths….every hour.

At last I am cleared for surgery. To date I've seen the following doctors:

DOCTOR/FACILITY	TEST
Michael Faust	physical, endoscopy, colonoscopy
Park Avenue Radiology	CAT scan (no contrast dye)
New York University Hospital	CAT scan (with contrast dye)
Stu Garay	lung functions, blood
Bala Subramayan	sonogram
Peter Schlossberg	lung biopsy
Bruce Raphael	bone marrow specimen
Columbia Presbyterian Hospital	P.E.T. scan
Amy Pan	lymph node check

Carol Portlock	lymph node check and 2nd opinion
Felix Heller	breathing exam
Charles Gibson	breathing exam and lymph node check
Valerie Rusch	lymph node check
Sloan-Kettering Hospital	blood test, urinalysis, Electrocardiogram (EKG)

It's as if they're assessing all the collateral damage first, before they snoop around the main bombsite.

A Matter Of Music

On Monday I'm in Patchogue, Long Island, in the house my great aunt lived in and left to my siblings and me. It has a stone front and a log cabin back. I used to come here as a boy and set pennies down for flattening on the railroad tracks just behind the woods. The quiet, the barrenness of the trees, the still chilly air of early spring – they all suit me well. I'm hiding out, away from all the diagnostic machines, and the clearly uneasy people painfully trying to look reassuring, and the unending parade of others, live or on the telephone, asking me how I feel. My answer is this: I feel great. However, I have volunteered for a guaranteed-to-make-you-feel-shitty program, beginning this Thursday (only three more days!) after which I should slowly be feeling good again. My emotional state is somewhat akin to the Democratic Republic of the Congo (formerly Zaire): lots of crazy thoughts battling over a mineral rich piece of territory (my brain). I'm fine and I'm a wreck. I live each day like it's my last, then I chastise myself for thinking so morbidly. That's how I feel, this millisecond anyway. Partly cloudy with a high of fifty-three.

I walk around with my newly purchased Audubon Society Field Guide to North American Trees. I learn to identify spruce, and pine, and oak, and maple trees. I find out that my favorite tree out here, the biggest one of all, is called a catalpa. I can't wait until spring. I'd love to be out here in May:

a)   because it will mean I'm still alive.

b)   because I'd like to try to identify the trees from their flowers.

Right now I'm using their leaves and bark. Luke and his babysitter Collette are coming out by train today. Luke is always perfect for me when I need courage. Say I'm feeling worried, or down, or scared out of my mind? I just think of Luke and try to imagine him asking me things like: "So Dad. You're going to die because you were afraid of having the operation?" Or "You're not sure if the cancer is in your bone marrow because you don't want to get stuck with the needle?" I love my little guy – even my imaginary version of my little guy.

Today I'll mix the music I want to listen to before and during surgery. Studies have shown that it's remedial to listen to good music even while unconscious, which may explain why I, as a youth, often passed out at parties when I got too wasted instead of heading off to the quiet of my own home. For pure adrenaline, I might include Ice-T's banned "Cop Killer." I too, were I a cop, would want to flay Ice T and his band for this song, but since I'm just a live-and-let-live-free-market-consumer unit, I absolutely love the song and get quite the charge out of listening to it. I can just see me now – my chest wide open but my arms flailing, head pumping, and lips moving to "Fuck tha Police....Fuck tha Police" or "I'm a muthafuckin' Cop Killer," E.K.G. blipping off the screen, blood pressure rising, the whole surgical deal going haywire for four minutes and change.

Then again, I was thinking of John Coltrane's "My Favorite Things," or some proto-peace REM tune. Easy slicing music. WCUT-FM.

Or maybe something instrumental might be better. I definitely want to avoid any sort of random song lyric further freaking me out in the already freaky environs of the pre-op waiting area. It's gonna be weird enough without any music-to-life disparity. I muse about Blood, Sweat and Tears' "And When I Die" here in my living room, but I don't know how much sense of humor I'll have just before I go under, and then when I do go under, I don't want to find out there really is a God, with an even sicker sense of humor than me (presumably the all-powerful would be able to hear what's playing on my headphones, right?)

Hmmm….perhaps a little gospel music? Just in case.

Back from Long Island, I feel the reality of surgery sinking in. I spend a few hours in a fog but feel better after therapy. I call the surgeon's nurse and tell her to tell the anesthesiologists I don't want any Raplon. She says I'll have a chance to talk with the anesthesiologist on the day of, but I say tell him or her now so they show up with a back up. How glad am I to have worked as a producer all these years! My credo has always been to treat the simple and routine as if it were new and complex, because the familiar is where most fuck-ups occur. I remember reading once that something like 80% of car accidents happen within three blocks of a driver's own home, on the streets he drives the most frequently and feels he knows the best. The film biz is the same – people relax and then they begin to make mistakes.

Further unsettling me is the call to Portlock's office. We never had a face-to-face conversation along the lines of "I'm your patient. You're my doctor" because I only decided to be treated at MSKCC after meeting Rusch. Two weeks ago I called Portlock's office and told her nurse to let her know I would now be her patient. That's the last I heard from them.

Today I go: "I just figured I'd call to say, you know, I'm having surgery on Thursday so I guess I'll see you in the hospital right?" I cribbed that line from Dr. Raphael at NYU – after our last appointment (I saw him a whopping two times!) he said to me: "I'll see you in the hospital," figuring Heller would operate on me and so on.

Portlock's nurse goes: "She's away at a conference but I'm sure she's given all your info to your surgeon and *he's* up to speed with Dr. Portlock." And I go: "Um first of all, *he* is a *she*, so can I get, like, not the pat answer and maybe a phone call from Dr. Portlock?" The nurse goes: "What procedure are you having?" I go: "a lobectomy" and she goes: "Whoa!!" This type of distinctly unscientific exclamation is precisely what you don't want to hear from anyone at this point because it indicates some measure of surprise and right now, surprise is bad. Extremely bad. Human-error-causing-unnecessary-death-type bad.

I know deep down that I'm basically in my surgeon's care now anyway, and part of the reason I chose her is that she's highly specialized in cancer-related care, but still, I want Portlock on the same page with her and at this point I don't even feel like she's reading the same book. Or should I say "he" just to underline my point? Fuck!

So I wig out for a while. One really nice thing about NYU was that all the doctors were networked into my friend Steven, so my care was highly personalized. I got phone calls from my doctors "just to check in" and the like. It was fabulous. That's what I've lost, at least temporarily, in the trade-off.

To keep myself calm, I've taken to trying to visualize waking up from the surgery – drainage tube on my right, oxygen mask on my face, inflating tubes on my lower legs (to prevent clotting), catheter in my bladder, spinal tap in my back, morphine in my brain, but above all, ALIVE and AWAKE. Hard to breathe but only temporarily. My wife and/or Mom and/or my brother Andrew and/or Dad in my room. The tough part over, maybe a cameo from Doctor Rusch. A smile and a wisecrack. Some nurse teaching me how to use the "rescue shot" button on my morphine catheter. My room – kind of orange and cream color, anyway something towards the warmer end of the spectrum. The weekend coming up, my family off to their Passover seders. Me for once having a good excuse to miss it – Hallelujah! At least that – thank you cancer! And speaking of which – a cancer-free body again. "What's wrong with me? Nothing. Just recovering from an operation, but after that, I'm good." Find something else to worry about dying of. Write a good story. Finish the movie I've been working on for three years. Go back to Splish Splash Water Park with Luke.

I'm still wondering what my final diagnosis will be once the pathologist has seen my whole tumor. But one thing at a time.... whatever else I may have, as far as I know I ain't got it yet.

Telling Luke

What am I supposed to tell Luke? When do I even tell him anything? How do I tell him? I remember when I was a kid and my mother was hospitalized with some problem (to this day I'm not quite sure what it was) and she was gone for a few days and then back and all right but the fear I felt is as palpable today as it was then. Where are you taking my mother? Why can't I go?

My first decision is to not tell anything to Luke until I know what the hell is going on. Since no one seems to be too clear about what the hell *is* going on for quite some time, it puts me in a serious bind. I'm sure he's got to be picking up on his kid-around-the-house radar that there are an awful lot of phone messages lately from people named Doctor So and So, coupled with the ubiquitous question asked of me by everyone hip to my plight, namely "How do you feel?" or its variant "Do you feel okay?" I've asked people to be careful not to leave any of the "We'll get through this" type messages on the machine. But I'm running out of time and I'm terrified he might learn about my illness from someone else, or worse, from some well-meaning individual saying something like: "You know Luke, no one lives forever."

I'm often stunned at the way people talk to children. I'm all in favor of honesty, but I recognize that children receive and process messages differently from adults. Tell them that someday we all must die and they envision a day in the not-too-distant future when EVERYONE will be dead, agonizingly so, including them. Tell them their father is sick and they will get terrified every time anyone else gets sick. They don't understand *degrees* of sickness like we do – the nuances of language are so frequently lost on kids – they're as literal as they come.

If I tell my son I have cancer, the next time he hears that someone died of cancer (which is inevitable) he'll panic. I ask my therapist about it and she gives me a great suggestion. She says: "Be honest. Be simple. Be brief. Then propose something fun like playing a game he enjoys." This is, in my opinion, some world-class advice. It actually might offset the refund I'm probably due from this very same therapist/marriage counselor since my marriage seems headed for divorce (a friend of mine says bluntly: "Probably due my ass. Tell her to give you your money back!")

I think there's a tendency for parents who have to deliver bad news to their kids to think of movies they've seen about death and illness; movies with surviving children. Or maybe it's just me and I'm projecting. In either case, you know the flicks I'm talking about. Dad's on bended knee. Little Bobby's wearing a tie wondering why Mommy isn't coming to the funeral and Dad's got to tell Little Bobby that it is actually Mommy's funeral they're going to, so she's coming, only in a "special" way. And the kid is sad but somehow understanding and of course the clincher is that the kid *is already prepared to articulate his feelings*. I see a lot of that shit in real life. Parents who want their kids to tell them how they feel right then and there.

Don't they watch sports on TV? Why do they think those immediate interviews right after the big game are all so idiotic? "You've just won the Super Bowl, how do you feel?" Sure, the guy will tell you he feels great, it was a team effort, and he was just trying to be all he could be, but what he figures out later, once he processes it all, is that he *feels* he was underpaid this year, or he *feels* he's entitled to some more recognition, or he *feels* his old man was wrong about him when he was a kid and now it's too late to show him because he died three years ago.

I'm not gonna ask Luke how he feels. Not for a while.

What I do is this: I wait until four days before I'm to go in the hospital. I tell him to come listen to me for a second. His babysitter Collette is nearby…I figure the less dramatic I am, the less frightening it will seem and telling him while someone else is around is a bit mellower. I tell him I've got to go to the hospital for a few days but I'll be back quickly. He asks why and I tell him I have something called a lesion inside of me (technically true, although later Steven the pediatrician thinks I may have caused him to imagine this lesion thing growing uncontrollably inside of me like a monster) and the doctor is going to take it out and that will be that. I tell him I don't know how I got the lesion but I'm not worried about it because the doctor said he could fix me up so it's no big deal. I tell him that he can come visit me in the hospital if he wants, just not the first day because those are the rules. Then I say, "Let's go get some ice cream."

And we do. Later I ask him if he's afraid because I'm going to the hospital and he says no and I say: "It's okay if you're afraid. But I wouldn't worry too much. Dad's gonna get fixed up just fine."

My guess is it's going to be a long time before he runs across the word lesion again. It just doesn't come up that much. I've never heard of anyone dying from a lesion although it's a daily occurrence among people with cancer. It's all about choice of words.

Just Me And A Couple Of Babes

April 5th, the appointed day, and I'm to be at the ominously named Memorial Hospital at 11 AM, with my procedure beginning at 1PM. Euphemistically speaking, my mass will be resected and then sent to pathology for full diagnosis. I'm gonna get there 15 minutes earlier so I can hang out with my Dad, since I'll be accompanied by my Mom and he wasn't up for the ride together. They had a bitter divorce about 20 years ago. I only wish I could watch their dynamic as they wait for me to come out of the operating room. Couples outside of divorce court, I'm told, begin to talk to each other like lovers again, so relieved are they to have their horrific divorces behind them at last. I'm not expecting anything within even the same solar system as that kind of reaction, but there's a vague hope my Mom will at least make eye contact with my Dad. I'd just like them to find a way to be comfortable exchanging niceties before they die.

I feel calm. I'm pretty good with facing inevitable situations, no matter how unpleasant. I mean I hope I'm not like one of those Auschwitz Jews who walked meekly into the gas chamber fully knowing he was going to die. Actually, I think I've finally managed to separate the idea of dying from my surgery. I've been trying to visualize waking up, seeing if I can prepare myself to be calm – or at least not panicky – when I see the plethora of equipment and find (possibly) a breathing tube down my throat in the recovery room. I went roller-blading yesterday to sort of reinforce to myself a very important truth, which is that life happens in small increments, moment to moment, and even when it appears to get highly dramatic, the way you live moment to moment will always be more important than what you do in extreme situations. Or put more succinctly, even if you beat cancer, you still have to get up and get your kids to school on time everyday. Heroism on a daily basis is the hardest kind. Today I'm going to be a hero to myself; brave, focused, and strong.

Had a great dinner last night with Layla, Mom, Steven and Kasino at a French place a few blocks from us. Restaurants that can turn out excellent food everyday impress me. Anybody can do it once, which sort of brings me back to what I was trying to say before. The discipline of excellence on a daily basis is a real achievement. I can't just fight through this surgery – I need to incorporate some of that heroism into my daily life in the time I have left on Planet Earth, which now seems to be a fair bit of time.

Maybe because I'm asymptomatic I'm still having an awfully hard time believing that I have cancer. With surgery I'll at least have some sort of physical hardship to associate with it, not that I wouldn't prefer to do without the whole illness/recovery package in the first place!

In other weirdness, it turns out my Dad's friend's wife is also having lung surgery today at MSKCC, by none other than Valerie Rusch. Together we can start a new trend in body art – "Lung by Valerie."

I wonder what this surgery will cost. I'm so lucky to be able to have this doubt. My insurance company, despite being an exploitative criminal organization engaged in massive fraud, will have to pick up the entire tab this time. MSKCC is signed up with my plan. More typical of my health plan was yesterday: I got five different health claims returned to me, each for the same specious reason that the membership identification number was incorrect. In each case, involving no less than three doctors, mind you, the ID number had been entered incorrectly, only each time it was a completely different number. I've never smoked crack, and I did after all attend college for four years, so what are the odds that I went to three doctors and each time entered a completely different number for myself which I was, by the way, *COPYING* from my membership card. Then of course, how do you explain the same doctor's office having two different incorrect membership numbers for me? Obviously the data was "mis-entered" by several of the health care thugs. Hence the real deal is "We won't pay your claim because the people who work for us are a bunch of knuckleheads." Why can't they just say that? Where's the shame in it? The Mafia serves a social function too, but you don't see them denying the illiteracy of their hit men.

Luke said last night he dreamed an African person with no clothes on crashed into his school with something like a baseball bat, only not a baseball bat, and me and Grandpa were watching, and Luke started to shout: "Emergency! Emergency!"

Chew on that one for a while. I asked him how he knew the person was from Africa and he said that the person said so. If this isn't anxiety about my upcoming hospital stay, then I'd better start monitoring his video watching and book reading more closely!

I check in on the ground floor along with about seven other people. Everyone looks nervous, which makes sense, because we're all about to have major surgery. I can't help thinking that we're not unlike a platoon of strangers who know that not all of us are going to make it out of the upcoming battle. Hopefully I'm wrong.

I'm brought to a cubicle to register, where I fill out a proxy form that authorizes Layla to discontinue life support in case something goes horribly wrong and I become a vegetable. She recoils when I tell her she's in charge of this, but you have to talk about it no matter how remote or distasteful it may be.

My wife, brother and I are shepherded up in an elevator, led down a hallway, and made to wait just outside a door that looks like the entrance to some kind of operating room. I can see big machines through the windows. The other patients who come up with us are all starting to get panicky, and I try to lighten the mood a bit by just being friendly. Saying hello. Wishing everyone good luck. I feel like if I can be fearless it will help the others, and since I'm a lot younger than everyone else, I am possessed by an odd sense of duty as if these were my parents or something.

Here's one for the dubious distinction list: I learn from a wall placard that on August 16th, 1948, George Herman "Babe" Ruth died in this hospital. Memorial Hospital. I believe he had cancer of the throat or esophagus. He also hit 714 more home runs than I, which helps reassure me that our fates at this hospital are not necessarily linked either.

My name is called and we move into the pre-op area, which is a series of beds with wraparound curtains that hang from the ceiling and form individual demarcations. The first nurse to enter takes my temperature as though I were a sick schoolboy about to be sent home for the day. But I understand that from now on, everything has to be monitored; heart rate, breathing, temperature, blood sugar, and so on. One technician comes in and inserts a catheter into my right hand, then, realizing she's missed the vein (my howl of pain is a good indicator) moves to my left hand and tries again, this time successfully. Someone else comes in and inserts my epidural catheter, but because my first blast of medicine is so strong, I only learn of this after I wake up from the temporary morphine slumber it causes.

A short woman looking to be in her mid-seventies enters. She is Sister Elaine, the hospital chaplain. She says she is here for spiritual guidance. She asks if I'd like her to say a prayer for me and I say: "why not?", figuring I've got nothing to lose. She says: "God is like a faithful trotting dog. No matter how you try to shake him, he just keeps following you around."

Soon I am deep in the land of Sedation. A team of husky looking young men walks up to my bed and uses an odd series of belts to shimmy me off the bed and onto another gurney. I say goodbye to my family and am wheeled through a series of long winding corridors. There are machines everywhere, but no people. Finally we reach the operating room, where an Asian Indian woman greets me. She is the most stunningly beautiful creature I have ever seen in my life. All I can see is her exquisite face, her luscious mouth, and her dark chocolate eyes; the rest of her is covered in green operating-room scrubs. I don't know who she is, or where she came from, but I begin to suspect that there's something fishy about seeing the most beautiful woman you've ever seen *right before you're about to have major surgery.* Am I going to wake up soon and see her in some celestial setting welcoming me to the afterlife? I actually feel myself wanting to get to know her, or find some way to contact her after my operation. It figures I'd find a woman like this at the very moment that I am hopeless to do anything about it. I can't very well ask her for her number. Or can I? My mind is actually formulating these thoughts. What should I say?

"I know this is completely insane, but I would really like to get to know you after my operation and I swear this is not the anesthesia talking."

Here I am waiting to have part of my lung removed, and *married* to boot, and still I am so bowled over by this woman's beauty that I begin to imagine a future together for us. It doesn't even dawn on me that I am wearing a plastic shower cap.

Maybe when they're finished with my lung, they can operate on my brain.

At last we enter the actual operating room, where I am hoisted onto a table covered in green sheeting. All of the machines around me are on wheels, and there are at least a dozen of them, which makes it feel like they just rigged this room together this morning. When I was a student in Italy years ago, we once visited the mythical operating "theatre" at the University of Padua, where some of the first surgical operations ever were performed. The room was literally a theatre in the round, with concentric rings of wooden benches sinking from the rafters down to a wooden plank in the middle of the room where the patients were laid down and sedated with ether. The operating theatre was built atop the Po River, so that the patient's blood could drain directly into the flowing currents. While surgery itself was gruesome and primitive, the theatre it took place in was possessed of a certain ordered majesty. Memorial Sloan-Kettering, by contrast, feels a bit like the kitchen of a Denny's restaurant, with vents and ducts and moveable machinery.

Several minutes pass before Dr. Rusch arrives. I keep thinking that I want to tell her I know another one of her patients from today. It's a terribly boring anecdote, even to me, but it's the closest I can come to holding a thought, given all the drugs I've had thus far. I guess I just want to tell her something – anything – to stress the humanity of the inhabitant of the body she's about to cut open. She walks in dressed in dark blue scrubs (I somehow expected a lighter baby blue), says a brief hello, and takes a quick look around the room. I start to tell her the anecdote, and she quickly cuts me off and says: "Let's save that story for after the operation."

If this turns out to be the last thing that anyone ever says to me, I'm gonna be really pissed.

One-Way Street

The first thing I see when I come-to after surgery is the Indian Beauty, again, leaning over my face as I am being wheeled into the recovery area, and saying to me "the operation went extremely well." She is not a ghost after all, but thankfully, for the first time in my life since I turned thirteen, I am so overcome with the euphoria of survival and the after-effects of anesthesia that I do not try to put the moves on her. I just smile politely.

But surgery is over! And Doctor Rusch – the Michael Jordan of thoracic surgery – has pulled it off with the thoracoscopy! I can't see my small incisions, but for once my morbid curiosity doesn't give a damn.

I learn that my tumor was on the bottom part of the upper lobe of my lung, so I got what's called a "wedge" resection, about an inch and a half by an inch and a half in size. My middle lobe is just missing a piece of its roof.

A quick check of me reveals:

1. An epidural catheter pumping morphine through my spine

2. A catheter in my left hand hooked into some glucose solution and a recent supply of Toridol anti-inflammatory goop

3. Foley catheter hooked up to my bladder via my dick

4. A blood drainage tube hanging out of me, unseen, beneath the bandages covering my incisions but definitely connected to a tube in my lung

Treatment is a funny thing. It is constructed like an onion. The more layers you peel away from the expression "We can treat you" in order to understand what treatment really involves, the larger and more frighteningly it begins to loom. In the distance, treatment shines like a radiant beacon of hope. As it approaches, it is all warts and blemishes. Only when you're finally ready to receive your therapy, be it chemo, or radiation, or surgery – only then do you truly understand what's involved. It's for this very reason that a good deal of my strategy is based upon not learning about anything that I may possibly avoid undergoing. If I need horror, I can go out and rent *Schindler's List*. When Doctor Raphael first suggests that my treatment will involve surgery I know there'll be some sort of cutting instrument involved. Then out of necessity I am briefed on a few more intricacies, such as the delights of having a chest tube for blood drainage post-op, and then further on I learn from the anesthesiologist that I'll be having a spinal tap inserted for pain management, and then from a nurse I learn I'll be rigged with a Foley catheter through which I can drain my bladder. They save these types of gruesome details for the days leading up to your operation, sometimes even the minutes leading up to your operation – when it's already too late to turn back.

For instance, I know little about chemotherapy, and even less about radiation. Right now they sound to me like variations on surgery that can potentially rid a person of cancer, or at least fight it off for a while. In other words, good. This is because I've protected myself from knowing the details until I absolutely need to.

But I've obsessed about the chest tube. What will it feel like? Will it look totally freaky to have a rubber hose hanging out of me? Then when I awake from surgery and see that the chest tube is pretty much concealed by a pile of white bandages, I switch my obsessing to the Foley catheter.

If ever there were a one-way street in the world, it is that narrow passageway which leads out...I repeat OUT...of a penis. Don't even think about putting anything *in* there because not only does it make me cringe, in some mystical way it makes every man on the planet cringe. We men may be pig-headed and ignorant and even downright stupid, but even the most pig-headed, ignorant and stupidest of us knows not to let anything *in* through that hole. Need to probe our rear ends with, say, a piece of tropical fruit? Fine. Need us to swallow live ants for prize money? No problema. Need to jab a Q-tip in our ear? Done. But the minute you want to invade the space reserved for the expurgation of our pee and sperm, you are crossing the male equivalent of the Berlin Wall.

So what then, I wonder, is this tube doing sticking out of my dick? How will I ever walk, or even more difficult to answer, how am I supposed to think about ANYTHING ELSE??!! Glad they at least waited until I was unconscious before inserting such a horrific device, though the mere fact of this catheter's insertion implies, *ipso facto*, that someday it is going to have to come back out of me. How does that work?

Once I'm up and walking around the ward, it occurs to me that more than ever before in my life, I'm being led around by my dick, something I'd foolishly hoped might end with adolescence. So much for high hopes. There's a tiny bit of play in the apparatus, so I can partially avoid the weird burning sensation of tube on *sensitive-as-hell* skin if I can just walk without any sway in my hips. Like Frankenstein.

Urinating comes about in reverse as well. I of course don't pee into myself, but there seems to be a suction effect working from the outside in, so it feels like all I need to do is not hold back and the urine will show itself out and into the drainage bag tied to my IV pole. Would an instruction manual be asking too much?

I get my first taste of Gel Treat lemon-lime-gel-type dessert, made by KOZY SHACK. It's Kosher for Passover too. Hey – I'm alive – I'll eat anything.

Incidentally, my back feels like someone left their sword in it.

I seem to sleep one hour at a time. Up at 2, 2:45, 4 something, and now 5:30. I dream I am in my office with my assistant Stephanie showing her how great my surgery went, dancing a few steps, and then suddenly I realize I've forgotten about my Pneumo-Evac drainage tube. There is blood on the floor, and the seal from the tube to the hose is damaged. I call the hospital to try to set up an appointment with Dr. Rusch. Then I gather up the bloody tube, go into the bathroom and begin washing it as well as some other weird apparatus resembling a sprinkler.

By now though, two guys semi-unknown to me – i.e. I think I recognize them but I don't know for sure – have come to the office and they're hassling Stephanie over some something that they're selling. I tell them that this is not a good time; Christ my hands are full of bloody surgical tubing, but they insist on staying and talking. I get belligerent and tell them to fuck the fuck off (these guys obviously represent phone solicitors who Stephanie's recently been too kind to and who I usually tell her to just hang up on, with no explanation.)

Back to reality. I'm about to call the nurse and ask for more morphine. I'm really sore right now, my bladder is full, but I don't understand muscularly how to piss through my catheter.

My roommate, an elderly Asian man, had his last bowel movement yesterday. It was diarrhea, which sounds like an even funnier word when mispronounced by a speaker of Asian languages. He and I have not yet spoken – I glean these details from overhearing his interview with his nurse. One of the joys of a semi-private room. And incidentally, what's semi about it? That it's not a public arena? More on my roommate – he vomited this morning. Mostly water – not the scrambled eggs he ate. When it came out it was the color of water. Somebody get me out of here as fast as possible.

I am able to get out of my hospital bed and into a chair by about 7AM. Have to up my morphine intake just for that. I have all my bags and tubes and wires hooked to a small trolley, which I wheel around the ward at a snail's pace. But moving nonetheless. All of a sudden I start to feel well.

I'm wheeled down to another floor for a chest X-ray, where I briefly chat with Andrea – pretty eyes and face, red bandanna holding up the remains of a chemo'ed head of hair – and get her story. Her breast cancer had spread to her lungs. Unusual as it was, Dr. Rusch decided to operate on both of her lungs at the same time. She's been in MSKCC for 10 days and is getting out today. Andrea is around my age and has two kids. I tell her I've got a kid too. We smile at each other, but it's not the happy smile of people thinking about how lucky they are to have kids. It's the hide-behind type of smile that means: "I'll do anything not to lose them."

When cancer patients say goodbye to each other, they always say "good luck." It seems like the only appropriate greeting for victims of a disease that strikes and spreads as randomly as this one. Old, young, strong, infirm, smoker, non-smoker, healthy, slovenly – cancer doesn't give a fuck, although it definitely loves people who hang out near dangerous chemicals like smokers and asbestos workers. Good luck means I hope you don't wake up any time soon feeling tired, or feeling a large bump near your lymph nodes, or in your neck. Good luck means work hard, love yourself, drink in your life and the people you love, struggle for me and I'll struggle for you, and let's see if this time we can catch a good break. Let's hope all our fight and goodwill isn't spat upon by our destiny.

Up on the ward, I go for another stroll, just after my respiratory specialist serves me up a ten-minute dose on a nebulizer. It feels like deep-breathing Vicks Vapo Rub. There's still no sign of my breakfast, or anyone from my family. My new Korean nurse Kin, "with an "N", introduces herself. She seems overworked already and pretty frustrated about me being food-less. I call my Mom and tell her to pick up some miso soup and hightail it uptown. She arrives an hour later and I practically dive into the Styrofoam cup.

Later my wife brings me a drawing from our son of a red cross on which he's written, "Dear Dad, I have a missing tooth! Love, Luke." Not "How do you feel?" or "I miss you so much" or "Get well soon". He wants me to know that the tooth fairy's on her way, which to me means, life is going on for this kid as it should.

Soon I get word that I'm being discharged. One of Dr. Rusch's assistants pulls out my chest tube. Painlessly. Weird, for sure, but painless. Kin comes in to pull out my bladder catheter, which she says won't hurt at all. I fall for the ruse and of course it burns like hell, but only for a minute or so. Any women out there who've had their gynecologist put an ice cold speculum inside them, I've got news for you….we're even. Oh how I wish I could erase from my memory the image of my poor shriveled penis with that orange tube sticking out of it. It's an image I could have used when I was a teenager and had to fight off premature ejaculation. Back then, my standard operating procedure was to imagine I was making love to this one particularly dowdy administrative assistant at my school, which usually bought me a minute or so of precious time. World War Two was a useful standby too. Who knew from catheters?

Without my even realizing it, my epidural morphine catheter gets yanked from my back, and then last of all my painkiller/anti-inflammatory/glucose/anything-else-to-pump-in-me catheter comes out of my left hand and I'm a free man.

On the way down the escalator, I see a guy in a New York Jets sweatshirt who is familiar to me though I'm not sure why. Didn't he bring his wife in yesterday? All I know is I recognize him from the hospital. I flash him a thumbs up and he shakes a way-to-go fist at me. I return the fist salute. There is so much pain and determination and fear written on his face and in his tightly pursed lips and I know in that moment that I am giving him hope in his struggle. I feel ennobled; so proud of myself, so happy to be getting out, yet somehow deeply bound to this stranger and his hurt. I feel like I'm fighting for someone other than my family and myself.

If this is not a miracle, then we may as well discard the word miracle altogether. Twenty-three hours after my surgery ends, I walk out of the hospital and take a car service home through a delicious spring rain. No one seems to like the weather except me.

Everybody's Got Something

I remember a Dashiell Hammett parable. A happy man with a family and the various trappings of a happy life walks to work one day, just like always, when suddenly a brick falls right in front of him, missing his head by inches before smashing to pieces on the pavement. He looks up and sees that the brick fell some fifty stories, with more than enough force to have killed him had he been walking the tiniest bit faster.

That night the man vanishes. He never makes it to work that day and no one knows what's become of him. The mystery lasts eight years until one day an old friend of his runs into him in another distant part of the country. The man tells him the story of the falling brick and how he realized right then and there how narrowly he'd escaped death. He then took the decision to leave his entire life of comfort and harmony and he set out to "make something of himself."

"What have you become then?" his friend asks. "Well, I've remarried. I have new children. And I'm doing the same job, only with a new firm."

I too am beginning to ask myself: "What do I do now that I've survived?"

One can't-miss approach would be to lead a healthier life (diet and exercise) and be more honest with myself about myself and somehow build upon the fortitude I've mustered for the cancer battle into the overall struggle known as Me versus The Unfilfilling Life. I decide to give myself twelve months to figure it out psychologically. By then I should have a good comfortable distance between myself and the world of lymphoma, plus I have this sense that a year is the minimum time a person needs to mentally adjust to trauma. Physically I'm adjusting at an absurdly fast pace.

I have my follow up visit with Dr. Rusch eight days after my operation. I surf on the computer in the Admiral's Club while I wait to be seen. The Admiral's Club has full Internet access, but I decide to stick to lymphoma-related sites only, even though a little devil on my shoulder wants to know if it's possible to download pornography, especially on such a fast connection. I assume they've blocked sites like www.girlsgonewild.com, although maybe the I.T. guy at MSKCC has a sense of humor, or decency, and figures "what the hell, the guy's probably got cancer, let him surf the porno sites if he wants to." But like I said, I'm going to stick to lymphoma sites only.

Just before seeing Dr. Rusch I get a chest X-ray on the 8th floor, then watch it magically pop up on the computer screen. MSKCC is all digital, meaning they don't use film for X-rays. The images pop up on screen and are then e-mailed to the appropriate doctor's office. I'm expecting to see a missing chunk somewhere on the picture of my right lung, about the size of a golden retriever bite. Instead I'm unable to see any difference in the two lungs. I ask the technician which is the spot where I had the surgery and he looks at the X-ray, perplexed, and says: "You had surgery?"

Up in Rusch's office, I get my preliminary exam from Christine, the girl who pulled out my chest tube in the hospital. She uses some alcohol-tinged cloths to remove some of the gunk still remaining from my bandage last week, then shares with me that she's had open heart surgery in the past, but was lucky enough to have her intervention done laterally, rather than cracking through her breastbone, which means she can still wear V-neck shirts. Me, I'm thinking, how many bazillions of people are out there who've been through the my-body-doesn't-work ordeal like me? It's as though you're completely healthy "like most of the world", at least that's what you think, and then something goes wrong, breaks down, and you find out you've got endless company. It seems everybody's got *something*. These are the broken down bodies that evolution designed for childbirth instead of cocktail parties, for rapid demise instead of eternal youth. Yet I, and Christine, and all the other survivors... we got a second chance. For Americans, who've never had a war on their home turf since the mid 1860s, this is as close as it gets to exchanging war stories. They call it the War on Cancer, on TV anyway.

Exit Christine. Enter Valerie Rusch. Since she kind of chafed at my pathetic, morphine-addled attempt to hug her in the hospital, I try something more dignified: I give her a card. I found a card reading: "Thanks a lot for coming to my rescue. You're like the cavalry, only you smell better." She doesn't open the card in front of me, but I can see she likes the gesture. I ask her when I can rollerblade again and she says I can do whatever I want. You can put a fork in me because, baby, I'm done. The same for my incentive spirometer breathing apparatus. It's a souvenir now.

I am ecstatic, but before I go popping the cork on the champagne, I've got to show up for a Tuesday appointment with Portlock. My pathology so far, in lieu of further stains to be processed, is small cell non-Hodgkin's lymphoma. I can't remember if that's the slow growing indolent MALT type, but I'm not gonna stress it until I get the full deal on Tuesday. Cancer provides plenty of opportunity to wig out; actually, it'd be pretty easy to lose your mind at any given moment if you chose to, but I'm sticking to my solemn vow for now: Just Say No to Freaking Out. But just for fun, this is one way the scenario could play out:

I see Portlock and it turns out I've got the aggressive type of lymphoma. So now I get chemo. Several weeks of long I.V.'s, probable hair loss (and that means all hair....from the curls covering your pubic bone to those annoying little hairlets in your ear), vomiting, major fatigue, a useless dick, a job I'm unable to return to, my business near to folding. Then say, six months from now, I get another tumor. Just a small one this time, but it's right back on my lung again. So it's surgery again, only this time no luck with the video thoracoscopy. Or maybe it's two tumors, one on each lung.

See what I mean? You don't really have to invent anything, just select your pieces and assemble to make your own gloomy puzzle.

Last night I had a strange and lovely dream involving Rusch and several of my friends. What I recall is being in an apartment, Rusch like a new pal hanging out with some of my old friends, me being clearly the center of attention. It was this wonderful me-centered ego trip. I felt so loved and cared for and safe. Protected by love.

I've decided to send a note to Felix Heller to let him know that I had my operation thoracoscopically; a procedure he never so much as mentioned to me. Maybe it will give him pause the next time a patient in a similar bind as mine comes in. Kind of hard for me to believe he never mentioned it, but I guess (or rather I would hope) that whereas Rusch thought success unlikely, he must have presumed it impossible and didn't bother to even bring it up.

Luke and I bought a couple of baseball mitts, a ball, and a bat today, and carried out an American ritual – the father/son catch. Felt like a dream come true.

A week later I read that Joey Ramone of the proto-punk band The Ramones dies. His cause of death – lymphatic cancer. He was 49, and according to his obituary he'd been fighting cancer since 1995. Also Stephen Prokopoff, 71, a "curator with an eye for neglected art," succumbed to non-Hodgkins lymphoma yesterday.

I don't know why I read the obituaries, especially because I'm specifically looking for people dying of lymphoma. Okay, I do know why I read them...it gives me a chance to say to myself "that's not me" but really it just scares the shit out of me in the end. Each time I see lymphoma listed as the cause of death I feel an adrenaline burst course down my spine – a brief, powerful shock of fear. Considering how good I've been about staying focused on my condition only, while blocking out all other not-specific-to-me detritus, why can't I stop carrying on this morbid, clearly non-constructive ritual? What's particularly frightening is that usually I find someone who'd died of lymphoma even though I only read the "celebrity" obits. There are hundreds of other deaths listed that I ignore.

I think for the first time in my life I'm acknowledging that I'm going to die someday. Really accepting my eventual death, not just spewing false platitudes about how I will die, and truly facing this idea means feeling sorrow, and anger, and fear about it. Right now I'm mostly angry and afraid. Plus for the first time I feel as though I am surrounded by death. Maybe I need to spend some time in a maternity ward to remind myself of how much life is arriving to replace humanity's unending depletion. I'm so acutely tuned in to cancer and sickness and death that it seems every other radio report, or advertisement, or newspaper article is about one cancerous malady or the other. I hear this almost non-stop cacophony of "cancer related, cancer causing, fight against cancer, cure for cancer, cancer foundation, carcinogenic, new testing for breast, stomach, liver, brain cancer." And on and on.

Today I am wondering if indeed I'm gonna get out of this fight so physically unscathed, or am I instead headed for chemo. I hope Portlock will reprise her "blip on the radar of my life" theory of my illness tomorrow, although, in any event, it's still time for me to really inform myself thoroughly about whatever my final diagnosis is, with the comfort of knowing that right now, my cancer has been effectively removed from my body.

So....How Did I Get Here?

April 17 – Full house at Dr. Portlock's office. Some so–called computer glitch left me off the appointment list, which means I'm likely to be in for a wait. I may have to give blood, though I'm considering just carrying around my own vial from now on and doling it out whenever requested. Not quite the splendor of the Admiral's Club up here on 67th Street. Muzak on the stereo, gray industrial carpet, a mix of cheap green leather, wine colored cloth chairs and love seats – still in the airline motif but more that of a bygone, low fashion era. It's the Lymphoma Lounge, where all the doctors are lymphoma specialists. Fluorescent overhead lighting through a faux asbestos grid of ceiling tiles. Don't they realize that fluorescent light has a green hue to it, which makes sick people look even sicker? Just a thought.

In any event, it feels a lot safer here at the Lounge now that my tumor lives in a laboratory somewhere in the Greater New York area.

After an hour wait I see Portlock. She looks younger and more fetching without her white lab coat on. I tell her I'm back to rollerblading (per Rusch's okay) and she tells me of a Kamikaze skater she saw going backwards, at night, down the middle of Second Avenue. A guy who, unlike me, didn't just finish a battle with lymphoma and still feels life is cheap. Especially his own.

She checks out my scars, which are improbably tiny in relation to the trauma they represent. She says: "We'll see you in six months. You're fine but you need to be monitored." I go through my litany of questions I've written and prepared for her, per a book I browsed in Barnes and Noble called "The Cancer Workbook" in which there was a checklist of "positive activities;" one of them being "I make lists of questions for my oncologist." One other memorable one was "I don't think about what caused my cancer."

There's a huge one. What the hell *did* cause my cancer? The conundrum is that you don't want to think about it because you don't want to get into a blame game with yourself, only you don't want to get your cancer again and you need to find some means of prevention. It's rarely as cut and dried as, say, just moving away from the nuclear waste dump you're living atop, or quitting smoking.

What causes cancer? Well, heredity, for one, which is reason enough not to spend much time thinking about what caused your cancer. You can't change your heredity. Some people are more genetically prone to cancer than others. Family history is the first thing your doctor wants to know about when he or she interviews you. I have no history of lymphoma in my family but that can be very deceptive. My mother's father died of a heart attack. Her mother died of lung cancer, likely brought on by cigarette smoking. How do I know neither of them had lymphoma? No one did an autopsy. It's quite possible my grandfather had lymphoma and didn't know it. Or what about his father and mother? I don't know what they died of, and I'm probably like a lot of people who don't know what their great-grandparents died of. Did they even know what lymphoma *was* back then? If you get hit by a bus and die, no one needs to do an autopsy, so how can we know you didn't have lymphoma, or some other type of cancer? Just look at me – I have lymphoma yet still I have no visible symptoms.

The booklet from the Cure for Lymphoma Foundation says this about non-Hodgkins lymphoma (NHL):

Causes & Types: Many factors may contribute to NHL, including heredity, viruses, and immune system deficiencies, but the exact causes remain unknown.

I've had friends tell me I need to eat whole cloves of garlic. I've had friends tell me I need to cleanse myself spiritually. I've had friends say I need to give something back to the world.

Instead I worship broccoli. I find comfort in the notion that cancer is broccoli-related, or rather, broccoli-deficiency related. I fantasize about living in a world where one day the simple consumption of this vegetable will lead to an end to the cancer plague. I can't remember where I read that eating broccoli is anti-carcinogenic but for some reason it resonated with me. Broccoli is a cruciferous vegetable, which means it belongs to the mustard family of vegetables, and Webster's defines that as: "any of several herbs (genus *Brassica* of the family Crucifere, the mustard family) with lyrately lobed leaves, yellow flowers, and beaked pods."

Lyrately lobed leaves? If I were sleeping with my broccoli, that's how I would flatter it: "Your lovely leaves are lobed like lyres." Okay, so her flowers aren't quite yellow, and her beaked pod is a bit awkward, but she's got some beautiful microbial agents, which can free me from my illness. Or at least prevent it. Or....which is the reality I'm afraid of.....at least allow me to *think* that broccoli prevents lymphoma.

I had a back injury once. I was 22 and one day as I was getting into a car in the middle of a cross- country NY-California drive, my back went out and I was in so much agony that I couldn't bend down far enough to get myself back in the car. The car was one of those low-slung jobs, a Triumph TR6 or something similar. This was in 1982. My friend and I were in South Carolina, and I had no choice but to just lie down on the side of the highway and try not to move. I figured the pain would pass soon enough. About an hour later, a South Carolina state trooper with a wide brim on his hat and a generally poor opinion of most of humanity pulled up and asked me what the hell I was doing. He forced me to get back into the car, and I screamed all the way as we drove to the nearest hospital. The doctors there gave me muscle relaxants and soon enough my pain subsided to a point where I could get back into the car again and continue our trip.

But the pain didn't go away for almost two years. Each day it varied from excruciating to dull, but it never ever went away in all that time. I went to a chiropractor, who told me I had a curvature of the spine. He treated me for a few months, then I went to an acupuncturist who stuck me with needles, and who actually made me feel better when we were together chatting, but the pain would come right back as soon as I would leave his office. I went to an orthopedist who told me to take aspirin every day. I went to another orthopedist who was the team doctor of the Los Angeles Lakers basketball team. He laid me down on the same X-Ray table he used for the then-Laker stars Kareem Abdul Jabbar and Earvin "Magic" Johnson. The table was about ten feet long, and it made me realize I would never dunk a basketball in my life. The doctor put my X-ray up on a light table and showed me where I had "a chip out of a vertebrae...a genetic problem," he said...and he prescribed a series of exercises for me to do each day. I did them religiously, and they definitely seemed to help.

Only the pain was still there. By now I'd given up playing basketball, and taking long walks, and doing activities that required me to stay on my feet too long (like going to museums). I'd kind of resigned myself to enduring some sort of back pain for the rest of my life. At age 24.

Then (and this is the part that sounds like a late-night infomercial) I had to pick up my elderly Aunt Blanche from her winter home in Florida, and I happened upon an article in the In Flight magazine about back pain. There was a doctor (I've since learned his name is Sarno) who was treating back pain as a stress-related disorder, in which the only remedy was stress and fear management. The idea was this: some people deal with stress by "locating it" in their backs.

Once the pain starts, it causes its victims to begin limiting the stress relieving activities they do (such as playing sports, or going on long walks) because they become afraid of the pain re-occurring and think these "physical" activities are likely to bring the pain on.

The treatment he advocates is to actively manage your stress, not be intimidated by your fear (in other words be brave – have fear but act in spite of it), and accept the pain as something caused by psychological factors only.

One week after I read this article and gave this seemingly nutty idea a try, my pain went away. It's been gone ever since.

As a result of this episode in my life, I began to believe in a connection between mind and body. I believe the mind can be healed, and in so doing, the body will often follow. So naturally I ask myself "what of my outlook, my way of life, my way of being could be causing the cancer? Am I hiding a murderous secret? Am I too wrapped up in myself? Is this where I've sent the stress in my life – from my back to my lungs?"

I wish I could say I believe that I am able to heal my cancer, but I don't. However, I think to some degree I can heal myself. I have pain I need to learn to deal with better. I have stress (and if I didn't before, I sure as hell do now). I have a brain poisoned with wrong ideas about me and the world around me. I believe in myself too little and I also let myself off the hook too easily. Look, I'll save the litany of my faults for the next magnum opus. My point is just that I'm imperfect and I could definitely use some fixing. This is how I see my role right now; fixer of me, eater of broccoli.

Other questions on my list today are:

–What's doing with experimental vaccines?

—Are my sudden cravings for sugar related to my lymphoma? (again, a little comic-book style bubble in the Workbook said "Did you know some cancer cells crave glucose?")

—What are the chances of recurrence?

Portlock lays it out for me clear and simple: vaccine experimental treatments are not for my kind of lymphoma and they're a long way from being ready anyway. My cravings for sugar are caused by something called a "sweet tooth." Totally unrelated to my cancer. Because I'm young, or more accurately, because I'm not 75, she can't tell me I'll never have to deal with this again. It could recur in 6 months, or 30 years, or never again. I ask about nutrition and she says "good cardio diet and exercise."

She ends our appointment by saying: "Stay healthy." For a moment I am shocked and then it hits me: I *am* healthy. Not just fine, or okay, or hanging in there, or as well as can be expected given the circumstances. I'm healthy. I'm a healthy 40 year old man able to do everything I could before – which I would have once joked means not much – but now means a lot more. We set a date for my next appointment: October 12th, the week of Columbus Day.

Naturally, through all this my more spiritual friends and my son's babysitter want to know if I believe in God or in some Force. But I don't. Sorry. I believe that God, were he to exist, ought to just go on television all over the world at the same time and say: "Can anyone else but a true divinity perform this trick?" God is supposedly everywhere at all times, so how tough could a worldwide simulcast be? I'm supposed to believe he can help the New York Giants win the Super Bowl, protect me from getting another tumor, and see that Li Chan Ming has a healthy baby in a mountain village of Northern Canton....all on the same day, mind you.....but he can't come up with a way to get himself on T.V.?? Please! My stepmother's been on the Home Shopping Channel eight times! Know what her ingenious entrée' into T.V. land was? Scented candles.

I believe I was very lucky and I also did a lot to help myself – staying calm, grieving at times, allowing my friends and family to help and support me (a HUGE impact there!), focusing on Luke. Whenever I'd get down or frightened I'd have the imaginary conversation with Luke about "Are you afraid to get your treatment, or to fight hard enough to survive?" and I'd say: "No. I'm not afraid and I'm not going to die. Yet." Which only meant "I am afraid, and uncomfortable, and uncertain, but that's not enough to keep me from wanting to be your Dad and to watch you grow up."

Back when I was seventeen, and I was having what I now suspect was a nervous breakdown, I used my kid brother and his unquestioning love for me as a sort of stepping stone back into my own fragile psyche. I still vividly recall driving with him around our San Francisco neighborhood, my mind as tenuous as oversized luggage on an overhead train rack, every moment feeling like a prelude to an irreversible trip into madness and panic. I recall hearing my brother Andrew's voice like an invitation to stay with the world, to remember him and us and the way that our bond mattered so much more than our parents' divorce, and my own despair about breaking up with my first-ever girlfriend, and the overwhelming fear I had of having lost my grip on life. Stay with me. Stay with this awful world because we have each other. I first began to heal myself then by thinking of my brother, spending more time with him, abandoning my fears and worries and just kind of hanging out in a kid's world and having a best friend who thought you were perfect just the way you were. My brother was all of nine years old at the time. What he was to me then, my son is to me now. Someone who only knows how to love me and ask for me and always be glad to see me.

Last night Steven called me at home. He said he'd been to see Faust for a check-up, and Faust sent him for a chest X-Ray.

"Steve?" I ask him. "Does Faust know why he sent *me* for a chest X-Ray? Did you ask him that?"

Steven goes: "No Michael. He doesn't know. He doesn't have any fucking idea why he sent you for a chest X-Ray."

Anyway, now he knows why he sent Steven.

Say It Ain't So, Joey

⚜

Date: Mon, 23 Apr 10:37:24 -0400

From: Michael <spark@inch.com>

Dear Friends and Family,

I know it's you that have been sending me those "Are You Horny?" messages, as well as "Get Discount Viagra Now!" Incidentally...yes and thanks.

Now for my news (yawn): I'm back at work. Oh fucking joy! Well anyway, it beats hanging out in a cancer hospital! My last check-up revealed that I'm in great shape. Now I've just got to be monitored every 6 months or so by my doctor, but my future looks good. My scars from surgery are pretty much healed and quite becoming if I do say so myself. Everyone I've shown them to has remarked: "Christ Mike, your belly is still huge."

Anyway, that was an eventful winter. I sure hope spring proves to be far, far duller. I crave dullness. I live for boring nothingness.

As you can see, little has changed, even though honestly, everything has changed....it's pretty weird. But fortunately, so am I.

Love love and more love.......Michael

My anxiety is back. I've been at some remove from my everyday, non-illness related life for a good three weeks, and on a psychological basis I'd say even more so — more like ten weeks. Suddenly my return to work is filling me with foreboding.

I'm back to my mercenary job making TV commercials. Fine, whatever, I need money and it's a high stress job. I should be able to just steel myself and get on with it. I sense that what's really frightening me is the pace. The constant availability by cellphone, the e-mail to read and return, phone messages, a social life, raising my son, all of it combined in a place where trees and open space are so scarce. And now the added responsibility of people depending on me instead of all this depending on others I've been doing lately. Actually, no, it's not that I've been so dependent on others, it's that I haven't allowed anyone to depend on me. It's been wonderfully liberating too. "Would love to do it, be there, help out, pay attention, call back…but I've got cancer and you know how that goes." For two months I had the world's best excuse.

My friend St. Clair Bourne calls. The conversation goes like this:

"Hi," I say.

"Hi."

"How you doing?"

"Nuts," St. Clair says. "Crazy story."

"Yeah. Me too."

"Real Crazy."

"Mine too."

"No Mike, I mean REAL CRAZY!"

"Me too."

"I'm talkin' Life and Death."

"Me too."

"I've got a brain tumor."

"Me too – only it's a lung tumor."

"Mine's benign."

"Mine's not."

"I'm getting radiation. Next month."

"I got surgery."

"Fuck man."

"Fuckin' A man."

I've changed. The world around me feels like a different place but I know it's just my point of view that's shifted. My friend Eleni's best friend died of breast cancer yesterday that had metastasized to her liver. I think: "That could easily have been me." It actually *was* me for three days, until the sonogram saw it as a kidney cyst.

The month of May begins with a freak out, as my brain seems to be stripped of its protective shell and suddenly it goes: "You might get cancer again and die like Joey Ramone! Holy shit!"

I pass by a line of eclectic fans and mourners outside CBGB's waiting to get in for the Joey Ramone tribute. My wig-out, or rather my near wig-out, is a bolt of fear that blasts through all my calm rationalizations about being out of the woods for now and hopefully forever. I can practically feel my legs melt beneath me. I quickly recover and switch my brain back to All's-Cool-It's-Over mode, but the truth is, I'm a long way from getting back to mental homeostasis. I still think about cancer every day, and just in case I get distracted and forget, there are loads of tiny reminders, like the late Joey Ramone, like my still-healing scars, like the medical bills that arrive in the mail, or my own morbid dilly dallying with the video footage I shot during the ordeal. Me at my pre-operation testing. Me having my temperature taken by a nurse. Me breathing into my spirometer. It's like I'm trying to remember and forget at the same time.

At the end of May I turn forty-one. I never once feel any of the dread you feel at getting older. I am honestly thrilled to have made it to this age! My birthday wish when I blow out the candle on my dessert at Restaurant Vong is this: 42.

And I'm sure next year I'll wish for 43. I really want to stay in the game now, come what may.

A History Of Weight

Maybe it's fatherhood, or midlife, or all the years I've gone without smoking cigarettes. I'm not the same guy I once was. I'm the fat version of that guy. The beer belly version. The version I vowed never to become.

It starts out as a fold. Two folds really, one on each side of my back about 4 inches up from my hips. The folds are the first sign I notice until I ask myself this precise scientific question: what is causing said folding to occur? That's when I realize that the hand rest in front of me is actually my stomach. I say hand rest because beginning about the time I was thirty-eight, I noticed that more and more people seemed to be unconsciously placing their hands on my stomach, which would have been all right if I were, say, James Bond on the phone with Headquarters in the middle of an international love tryst – my bed sheets unmade, my hair mussed in a still-attractive way, and lovely Svetlana the double-agent resting her hands on my prone, washboard abdomen. But unfortunately, the people who rest their hands on my stomach are all, like me, in a position known as standing up. And their hands aren't actually tired; rather, they are unwitting instruments of geometry idly describing the protrusion that my belly has become. Twenty pounds worth, to be exact. Twenty pounds on a body that's prided itself on being in the neighborhood of one hundred fifty five pounds since the end of puberty. Not only am I no longer in the neighborhood, I've moved to a whole new zip code.

I'm five foot nine, and like my father, I like to say that I'm not overweight. I'm just a little short for my weight. My father is six foot two, and very short for his weight. My sister is starting to become a midget for her weight, and my mother will tell you that she wouldn't mind growing a few inches taller herself. My half-sister and her Mom are only the latest editions to the ongoing saga in my family. Only my brother Andrew and I never had "girth issues." He is a tall, strapping, former river rafting guide. I am short and a weak swimmer, but I smoked cigarettes for two decades. When I finally quit smoking for good, just before Luke was born, I began to gain weight. Soon it became hard to tell which had been most responsible for my twenty-pound surge in corpulence: quitting smoking or the excesses of fatherhood. I eat tons of late-night chocolate and all the candy I can pilfer from Luke's toddler-year birthday parties, although even that only explains the how of the question, not the why.

I used to exercise. I'm sure it had a lot to do with my trim physique of yore. I would play pick-up basketball at Tompkins Square Park, or run the floor in a weekly game organized by a ticket-scalper acquaintance of mine up at a high school on 68th Street. We all pretty much sucked. Men playing basketball in their thirties and forties is not a pretty sight, unless you are an orthopedist in need of new patients, but the calorie burning was always a good reason to come back for more. To me, every game I played without re-spraining an ankle was its own small victory. Soon though, the personal victories began losing out to the stints on crutches, six-weeks at a time, unless I'd get lucky enough to twist my ankle near a Korean deli. In that case I'd have access to bags of ice, the swift application of which usually translated into a 2-week reduction in crutch time. I don't even want to get into how pathetic it is to mentally register the distance to the nearest Korean deli when you are about to play pick-up basketball. I haven't experienced sexual impotence, but I've got a hunch this is pretty close to what it feels like.

I started jogging regularly right after Luke was born. I'd run and listen to National Public Radio on my headphones. Programs like All Things Considered, or This American Life, or even Car Talk. Anything to distract me from the tedium of running. Layla went so far as to buy me a little Eddie Bauer calorie counter to encourage me. It was a complicated little device that hitched to my belt. I soon realized it had been designed to show why Eddie Bauer made his name in clothing instead of electronics. Part of it was my fault – I'd apparently mis-entered the length of stride data, and thus in my mind the miles were elapsing like ticks on a metronome, whereas the Eddie Thingy had more of a church bell rhythm to it. My two miles were equivalent to Eddie's zero point eight.

I stuck with it though. I'd run a lap around Washington Square Park, and tell myself that I'd just burned off the caloric equivalent of a Twix bar, or a Fruit Roll-Up (it's tragic, really, the things they give kids at birthday parties these days). Or I'd busy myself with imagining the total number of footsteps I'd taken in my life. I'm not quite sure where that idea came from, but it's an accurate indicator of just how boring I found running to be. Nonetheless, I persisted. After about a month, I was able to run without a radio, and my mind developed a lesser dependence on outrageous notions. I was proud of myself. I felt in control. I became the athletic person I'd once been as a youth.

Unfortunately, for the next four years, I continued to believe that was the case, even though my running obsession was really just a flirtation, at best. I believed I was in shape – "running shape" to be precise – and I dismissed the renewed, creeping expansion around my waist as probably just some sort of mix-up in my wardrobe. My memory developed a default setting whereby it always felt like I just went running four days ago, even though in the recesses of my mind I knew it'd been more like four weeks. Then four weeks became four months, and eventually four years. I wasn't part of the general exercise culture, nor did I have any medical impetus to revisit the issue of my extra weight when I had my first check-up with Faust. He told me I was "fine."

At home, Layla wasn't much of an athletic inspiration, to say the least. She acted as if Allah himself had inserted some sort of prohibition on exercise into the Koran, even though she isn't the slightest bit religious otherwise. She liked to tell me that we had just reached an age where folds are to be expected and enjoyed. It was actually a very lovely and mature notion on her part – at least my wife didn't mind the folds. I only truly became concerned about them when all the hand resting started up again.

During my lung ordeal, I wasn't about to start trying to lose weight. With a cancer diagnosis? Are you kidding me? Sudden weight loss is one of the signs you're supposed to look out for! Besides, why deprive myself then when it looked like I might be deprived of every good thing in my life, including my own existence? I kept eating. I didn't run at all. The closest I ever came to exercising was the rollerblading habit I started up over the summer. My legs got strong as hell, but I wasn't shedding any pounds.

But now things are different. It's the middle of June. I feel as healthy as I ever have, and I'd probably be thin as well if I could rollerblade all the way to, say, Pittsburgh on a daily basis. But I never go much further than the West Side Highway, which is about three hundred miles short of the Pennsylvania border. I wouldn't mind losing a few pounds but I'm really ambiguous about the whole thing, until the bottom drops out. The catalyst for change arrives in a decidedly non-medical sort of envelope. It's a letter from my oldest friend Gary, who lives in Los Angeles and who apparently uses his desk for a dumping ground, like I do. He's written a note on a Post-It that says:

"Dear Michael, I found this roll of film in my desk after fifteen years. Enjoy. Love, Gary"

The Post-it is attached to several black and white photographs that appear to have been taken in Paris. Outside Notre Dame. Inside Beaubourg. I quickly remember that the only time Gary and I had ever been in Paris together was indeed fifteen years ago. I was on my way to meet Layla for a vacation on the island of Cyprus. It was 1987 and civil war was raging through Layla's home town of Beirut, where she was doing research for her doctoral dissertation in anthropology. Since the welcome mat in Beirut for American guys named Solomon was a bit on the unwelcoming side (Terry Waite, the last guy to see the welcome mat, wound up a hostage for seven years), and the rest of the world wasn't exactly keen to embrace things (or people) Lebanese for fear they might explode, we agreed to spend a couple weeks vacation in Cyprus. It's only a ten-minute flight from Beirut, and it's been the scene of Turko/Greek enmity since 1974. Places caught up in their own U.N.-monitored troubles don't make a big fuss about who comes to visit. They just figure you're desperate, or a complete idiot. They're not far off actually, except that my plane also went via Paris, so I decided to stay a few days and take in the sights there too. Gary and his future wife Trula were headed to their friends' wedding in the south of France. We met, we embraced, and apparently Gary took pictures.

I instantly identify two distinct trends in the photographs. As a 26 year old, I had a lot of hair on my head, and very little flab around my midriff. As a 41 year old, I have the exact opposite in both departments. Monstrously so. In fact, it is abundantly clear that I am now a person who might answer to the moniker "Fat Pig." The hair I can't do anything about. I tried Rogaine for about three months, which may indeed have grown a few strands of my hair back, but at the cost of having a sulfuric acid sensation on my pate. I'd rather be bald than hollow.

Nevertheless, I resolve in that moment of reckoning with the photos to embark on my first ever diet. But I'm too lazy to read a book about what kind of diet to do, and I'm sure as hell not going to go see another fucking doctor. I can just see it:

"Hi Doc. I was wondering if you could give me some advice about a weight-loss diet?"

"Oh, you again. Say, why don't we check you for some more cancer while you're here?"

Fuck that.

So I try something that seems logical, and that I know is foolproof: I stop eating. I pretend that it's Yom Kippur (and that I still believe in God). I try to focus on the cleansing aspects of fasting, which works reasonably well until I start to get hungry. As in, very hungry. The day becomes a glacially slow trudge from one missed mealtime to the next. I can think of nothing other than food. I wake up and hunger for eggs and toast. I get to work and hunger for sushi and tuna melts. Since I've been eating like a pig for so long, I'm forced to endure a mid-afternoon hunger for the pork buns I used to get in Chinatown, before my evening hunger for steak tartare and ravioli sets in. The night is the most difficult. I am haunted by chocolate. Not just a little chocolate either. I want enough chocolate to make up for the calories I've been missing all day, which is what's known medically, I believe, as P.M.S. Day one of my diet is, in a word, torture.

But the next morning I am less hungry. I hop on the scale and see that I am already one pound lighter. I feel inspired. Only nineteen more days to go at this rate. I start to daydream about Bobby Sands, the Irish Republican Army prisoner who died in a hunger strike back in the 1980s. He fasted about sixty days before he succumbed. I was genuinely sad when he died; and yet today my deranged mind is wondering how much weight he lost. Why the hell are we so dependent on food anyway? Wouldn't our lives be much better if we only needed to eat, say, once a week? Just look at me – starving myself because I'm too vain to accept that I weigh more than I did when I was a youth. I feel like I should at least have a political cause to tie my absurd suffering to. I should probably call around and see if there are any meaningful hunger strikes going on that I can align myself with. After all, I'm already on day two. I could be useful to someone.

By 11 A.M. I decide to stop starving. I try another idea. Miso soup. I read about it somewhere – these hundred-year-old Japanese guys who say miso soup is the secret to their longevity. I vaguely recall one of my health-nut friends telling me you could live on miso soup alone. Since I've had nothing to eat for the past twenty-four hours, it makes sense that I introduce some of this soy life force into my diet immediately. I ask one of the women in my office to get it for me from the local health joint because I can already picture myself becoming enamored of a carob bar if I go myself. Why flirt with temptation? The soup unexpectedly arrives with free crackers, which causes me to have an epiphany about my diet. I say to myself: "Crackers don't make you fat unless you eat several dozen of them. You should learn to eat lighter on a regular basis." And so I decide to do two of the most un-American things I've ever done. I eat *less* and I exercise *more*. Half a sandwich. Half a plate of pasta. One bite of chocolate. I pretty much consume the same foods as always, only less of them. I ask for smaller portions of food at restaurants. And I start running a couple of times a week, for about twenty minutes each time. No particular schedule, no entry in my calendar to remind me…I just make myself do it twice within the week.

And within three weeks, I lose ten pounds. A month more, and I've lost all twenty.

Don't worry, I hate me too. People who lose weight easily, I know, deserve to be shot, but actually, I don't get off as easily as it seems.

Instead what happens is that I feel terrific and a lot of people start telling me that I look terrific, except there's something oddly disquieting about their compliments. They say: "You look great," but what I know they're saying is "You look great…for a cancer survivor." There's a deviously simple way to tell. No one ever asks me *why* I look so "good." I don't get: "Hey, you look great. Did you go on a diet or something?" Occasionally I get "Did you lose weight?" but no one follows it up with "How did you lose weight?" The assumption is that cancer did it to me.

Part of me wants to just say, "Yeah. It *was* the lymphoma," because I know that the person asking me may then have to think, even for just a nanosecond: "Gosh I wish I had cancer too." Trust me; I have mined the spiritual depths of vanity and I know of what I speak. When I thought I might be getting chemo, I actually looked forward, for one brief instant, to having such an admirable excuse for hair loss.

The more I think about it, the more my brain is becoming like TV — a couple of good programs surrounded by hundreds of channels of idiotic noise. Every day's a struggle to hang on to the remote. However, my runaway vanity notwithstanding, I'm pleased to have taken a positive step for my health and self-esteem. Though not necessarily in that order.

A Palatable Way To Go

I look down and I see my ankles. They are wrapped in a towel and connected to a 5-inch thick bungee cord. If I look past my ankles, all I can see is the surface of the mighty Zambezi River, 350 feet below me. On one side of me is the border of Zambia, and on the other is Zimbabwe. The bridge I am standing on connects these two countries, and presently, it is the only thing connecting me to the planet Earth. Suddenly three Zambian guys behind me shout: "Three, two, one, BUNGEE!!" and I dive up and out, as far as I can.

The world becomes silent. The chitchat on the bridge is no longer audible and the churning rapids of the river are well out of earshot. But in another millisecond or so, my upward momentum will be all used up and I will begin plummeting at warp speed back into the realm of sound until—I am told—the bungee cord around my ankles will snap taut and save me from a watery death below.

It's August and I am back in Africa. "Whose idea was this?" I wonder, referring to my sudden lack of terrestrial purchase. "Who decided that I should be in this particular place at this particular time?" "Am I here for entertainment, or to fulfill some higher purpose?" (That's the great thing about the mind. You can actually fit all those thoughts into an instant, even when airborne.) I tell myself I am totally fearless. I am thinking of the terminal patients who are grateful for the experience of having had cancer.

All right, maybe I'm a little frightened. And I'm also thinking about what it would look like to end up dead at the end of a broken bungee cord, smashed and scattered across the Zambezi River. Like I said earlier, I can't control what I think about, only what I think *of* what I think about.

But I really do think about the terminal patients. I too have been searching to find the so-called "gift;" something to take away from this experience other than just relief that its over or worry that it may come back. What the terminal patients are trying to say, I believe, is that not being afraid of the end of your life is a victory in itself. Your conquest is that you can at last accept, as the orator Robert Ingersoll once said, that this is a world "where Life and Death are equal kings." Few people die painlessly, or quickly. Cancer is a horrible way to go, however, it seems to have an uncanny knack for mining several fine attributes from its victims before doing away with them, such as honesty and courage and compassion. Although it is extremely difficult to deal with psychologically, this is something quite different from being mentally debilitating, which cancer rarely is. I'm beginning to understand that these patients are grateful for the chance to have examined their lives and perhaps made some changes, or mended some fences, before it was too late. Before they had to die the tragic death – the death of regret.

Hanging here in mid-air, about to plummet 350 feet or so, is not part of a gift of cancer but of survival. I probably am crazy to try a stunt like this, knowing that I've just been through the fight of my life for a son who is counting on me to raise him. But no one has ever been hurt here in ten years. What looks like an incredibly dangerous sport is actually safer than airplane travel. And the gift, if any, is inside of me, where I know what Luke's hair smells like when he comes out of the shower, and what his eyes look like just before he drops off to sleep, and the comfort he feels when he rests his head upon my shoulder. I'm paying attention to life far more than before. I'm trying to spend more time listening and less time talking (a HUGE endeavor for me, a kid who didn't speak until he was four and has been making up for lost time ever since). I'm contacting friends I've lost or let go of over the years, not because I'm suddenly nostalgic, but because I realize how much I've really missed them.

Some of my friends tell me: "Mike. You're turning into a chick."

As my body speed approaches two hundred miles an hour, I begin to seriously wonder when the bungee cord is going to engage. I've been in free fall a lot longer than I expected. I should be bouncing up and down by now. I should be laughing at the ecstasy of having survived the fall. I should be formulating how to describe this experience to my friends still up on the bridge, whom I should be seeing again, shortly. Instead, I am hurtling toward oblivion in a swimsuit.

But I'll be okay, right? I just need to make it past October.

Beirut, Sister City

My six-month checkup is only a month away and I'm thinking: "I'm gonna be fine." Portlock said back in April that I should think of this disease in terms of decades, but only a fool would believe that and not wonder why she wants to see me in six months. This is part of my burden. I need to keep thinking positively and optimistically and then behave as if the worst case might instead be true. Somewhere in this interaction lies a fundamental truth about life itself. Keep looking up but be prepared for everything to fall apart at any moment. Cancer patients are just more keenly aware of the tenuousness of existence. We have no choice but to live in the moment. It doesn't mean we do it better than anyone else. We just recognize it for what it is. Fleeting.

A few days later a couple of airplanes ram home a similar point. I'm driving home from the U.N. school where I've dropped Luke off and I'm going to Michael's house to pick up a bunch of DVDs I loaned him. He hands me the DVDs and says: "Turn on your radio. A plane just crashed into the World Trade Center." I say: "Get the fuck out of here." But he says he's serious. I tune to 1010 WINS and hear the stunned voice of John Montone, saying that one of the Twin Towers is on fire. In my mind's eye I see a small propeller plane, an image probably drawn from a photograph I've seen of the plane that hit the Empire State Building back in the Forties. But it's only a few more minutes before they announce that there are reports that a second plane has hit the other tower.

I round the corner of Second Avenue and 3rd Street and hear a collective scream from the crowd suddenly gathered there. I brake and get out and see that there are now two horrific fires burning before our eyes.

They are so far up that it is instantly clear that there is no way anyone could possibly put those fires out. How could you get enough water up that high?

A swirl of thoughts and emotions hits me and in an instant I recognize them as the same feelings I had when I got my diagnosis. I feel the rug being pulled out from under me again and I remember how this feels. I don't actually live the events in such a self-centered context – like everyone else I'm thinking What the Fuck is Going On, except that I also think to myself "Many people are dead or about to die and it looks like I won't be one of them this time." I stupidly consider heading downtown at this point, a decision that probably *would* get me killed, but I decide to head home, find Layla, and make plans to get Luke from school.

On our way to the school Layla turns to me and says: "Welcome to Beirut." In the 15 years that I've known Layla, I've heard Beirut bandied about a thousand times by others to describe disaster or semi-disaster situations. Indeed, Beirut is sort of the poster child for all things terrorist and destructive, but this is the first time Layla, who grew up in Beirut, has ever drawn a parallel to the former madness of her hometown. She is just the person you want to be with in this type of situation...she instinctively knows what to do. Grab the passports, get the kid (even I figured that one out), buy some water, and take along a small transistor radio.

At the school all the parents are leading their kids away. We tell Luke that there is an emergency because two airplanes crashed into the Twin Towers. Later on in the day, he tells a friend of his that smoke was coming from the World Trade Center. But it's not until the next morning, when he watches the image of the second plane exploding into the South tower, that his brain truly registers how serious things are. I am reminded of the words of the Mission Control operator when the Challenger space shuttle blew up. The sky was filled with that unforgettable white smoke cloud and the operator said simply: "Obviously, we have a major malfunction."

September 11th 2001 is a lot like what cancer feels like psychologically. To me. I'm not asking anyone to care, it's just that people are always asking me: "How do you feel?" and suddenly, courtesy of Al Qaeda, I have a decent explanation. I feel I've become a witness to a world I once felt a part of. In my brain I try to determine what to do, which way to go, where can I find some sort of solid foundation to guide me. And how can I possibly reduce the consequences. Where do I apply for parole, or a pardon, or whatever else gets you out of this mess and gives you a second chance, or a reprieve, or a break? How can I go back in time, and just shift the whole world into reverse for a few seconds so I can prepare and make a move?

A stream of ash-covered people in business attire comes marching up the Bowery. Many are dazed or in tears. I decide to go donate my blood, though I wonder if I'm still allowed to since I have, technically, a blood disease. I call the hospital and they say, as politely as they can, thanks but no thanks.

I feel polluted. The world is crumbling and I have cancer. Had cancer. May have cancer again. I realize I didn't survive to live in "this kind of world" or "that kind of world." I survived because it's in my nature to survive. I survived because in one world or another I have a son who needs me and who I need too. Once the illusion of immortality is shattered it never comes back. I am alive because I am not dead; it's as simple as that. What I do with my living breathing body and soul is totally unimportant to the moons of Jupiter or to the toppling buildings of Lower Manhattan. They are controlled by gravity, I am governed by death. But don't mistake me for some hero who is totally unafraid of death or suffering. I'm just more *aware* of its constant proximity. It's like I was born thinking I was on a boat, grew up seeing it as more of a life raft, and now I feel I'm just a fallen leaf that may or may not be swept under by the next wave. Landfall, in any event, is a total impossibility.

I'm a person.

A happy-to-be-alive person. A person who is less afraid to feel pain and more aware of how much pain courses through the lives of the people I see on the subway every day. Or the families of firemen, and brokers, and secretaries in tennis shoes.

The next day I go down to Ground Zero, where the towers used to be. The damage is truly massive. Television images, because they are restricted to the ground, don't give a good picture of the size of the area destroyed. Besides the two towers, the entire World Trade Center plaza is destroyed, and many adjacent buildings are going to have to be brought down or totally rebuilt, if they don't collapse on their own. Aside from all the ash and soot and metal covering blocks and blocks, there are billions of pieces of paper that have rained down in all directions, as if a bottomless filing cabinet had been emptied from the skies. A lot of what makes this situation so surreal is the way in which these objects and papers seem to reflect a moment frozen in time.

Two days later, September 13th, it is still so quiet that all I hear as I ride my bicycle past Washington Square Park (which is surrounded by New York University) is the whirr of the wind. Not even Christmas morning is this silent. Downtown below 14th Street is closed off. There are police roadblocks at 14th Street, Houston Street, and Canal Street. 99% of all businesses south of 14th are closed, the subway is closed, and there are no cars or buses down here either. We have taken to walking in the middle of the street simply because we can.

I see a typical New York City madman (long beard, matted hair, crazy dog) walk down the street with a sign saying "Bomb the Entire

Middle East. Fuck Allah. Kill the Bastards" and so on. It is reassuring to see that this person is obviously insane.

This whole disaster defies our need to quantify. How many dead? How many injured? How long will it take to restore and rebuild? All I can think is this: Be glad you're alive. Relish the hand you've been dealt. Play your cards well.

The Wisdom Of Gertrude Stein

For the next two and a half months, my neighborhood is redolent with the acrid smell of the fire. There is no end to the smoke wafting above the financial district. It has become an inverted landmark – a billowing suggestion of the fallen skyscrapers. Our local fire stations are draped in flowers and hand-drawn notes of condolence from children all over America. Someone keeps votive candles lit throughout the night and day. We take our kids to our neighborhood firehouse on Great Jones Street, where 10 out of 11 guys died in the collapse. Luke draws a picture of the two towers on fire and writes: "Thank you for saving the people."

I come home and find a note in the elevator saying that Timmy Haskell, a fireman who was dating a girl on the second floor of our building, is no longer alive. Both he and his brother were lost. One day he's the guy parked outside with the bright smile and the kind word – the next day he is gone. Later on I go to Timmy's fire station on Lafayette Street, where 11 out of 13 guys died, and one of the survivors tells me that Tim was a great cook who always got him to eat healthy food. If you know anything about firemen, you know that they eat most of their meals together. Everyone at the station and in the streets is wearing their shock, but no one seems to be able to absorb it and make any sense of it.

I do no better than anyone else. I try to focus on getting through each day, because I know that it will take time for the shock to wear off, the analysis to make sense, and the solution to become apparent. But right now I feel as if I am inhaling far more than I'm exhaling. Besides, I am trying to deal with another personal cataclysm as well.

Layla and I have decided to separate after sixteen years together, eleven as husband and wife. I need to find a new place to live. I have the distinct feeling that an attack like the one we've just lived through is the kind of earth-shaking event that will cause a lot of people to reassess their lives, and their loves, and make changes accordingly, but in my case, we'd already made the decision a month before the attacks, and I see no reason to go back just because the whole fucking world seems to be falling apart. I keep thinking of that Roy Liechtenstein painting where the woman in the business suit holds her head and moans: "Nuclear War? What about my career?" In my case it's "Thousands dead in Manhattan? What about my marriage?"

Gertrude Stein once said that death and taxes never come at a good time. The same can be said for cancer, terrorism, and divorce.

For the first five or so years of our marriage, our friends saw us as an "ideal" couple. We seemed suited for each other. Each of us loved to travel and spoke several foreign languages (my wife grew up tri-lingual in Beirut – French, Arabic, and English, to which she added Spanish, Italian, and German; I went abroad to study in college and learned Italian, French, and Spanish). We are both pretty smart (she could probably win a Nobel Prize if she wanted; I'm more likely to win a spelling bee) and we never seemed to run out of things to talk about. We both love to cook (she'd win the Iron Chef; I might win special mention in a pasta cook-off) and to eat. We would spend hours playing backgammon (Final score: 62,433 – 62,432, my favor), smoking cigarettes, and laughing at each other's wisecracks.

I remember before we got married, my father warned me that it would be tough to bridge our cultural differences. His second wife Sue is South African, and even though she's white and Jewish like he is, even they had their share of cultural-issue-related throwdowns. What might cause such a melee, you wonder? Well to begin with, there's the question of properly discarded olive pits. Layla and

I nearly broke up once because I put an olive pit I'd finished onto the tablecloth of the restaurant we were eating at, just next to my plate, instead of putting it on my plate or into an ashtray. I insisted that this was customary practice in great societies, such as Italy and Greece (I think I was wrong about this, actually) and she got so upset she seriously considered never seeing me again. As I said before, I didn't marry a nut, so why all the hullabaloo over an olive pit?

In Layla's mind, this was the type of behavioral breach that would indicate a hopeless situation. It was like: "The guy puts his olive pit on the table, next thing he'll be blowing bubbles with his spittle. Or wearing his napkin on his head. I can't marry a guy like that." She didn't see an olive pit per se, she saw a waste product emerging from a person's mouth. She saw a cultural educational chasm that was wide and unbridgeable. She saw, in sum, the person her mother had always warned her about.

I remember a woman who told me that she broke up with her boyfriend because he didn't know who the Jetsons were. The Jetsons – the cartoon family that lives in Outer Space. On the surface, it sounds ridiculous, but of course what she meant is that there were just too many gaps in upbringing for she and her guy to ever find meaningful communion with each other (her boyfriend was from Chad, or some country like that where the Jetsons aren't yet sold into syndication).

I always felt that Layla and I had enough in common to overcome whatever our differences were. I was wrong. An easy explanation is that parenthood changed everything, but I suspect that the roots of the conflict were established long before our son entered this world.

The reason it's so easy to "blame" parenthood is that it offers a virtual cornucopia of things to argue about. Here's a rough catalog of topics I thought I'd never be arguing about:

1. Can our son eat solid foods yet?

2. Is it time to toilet train him?

3. Should he be walking yet?

4. Is his bottle too hot?

5. Is his bottle too cold?

6. Is this the right bottle?

7. Should he wear a sweater?

8. Does he need a swimsuit?

9. Whose turn is it to have a break?

10. Should we take a bottle of water along with us?

11. Is the water too cold?

We argued about arguing. We argued about who started the arguing argument. We invented our own secret arguing code:

SURFACE STATEMENT	UNDERLYING MESSAGE
"I'm not raising my voice!"	I expect to lose this argument
"I'm not shouting!"	I expect _you_ to lose this argument
"I'm not screaming at the top of my lungs!"	I'm really, truly not raising my voice! (see above)

Often I'd find myself having an argument with Layla when she wasn't even there. The voice inside my head would just pick up on the topic and construct a winning series of thrusts and parries in my imagination. I hated myself when this happened, and believe me, it happened a lot.

We'd almost never argued before we became parents. Now we couldn't stop arguing about everything. Our friends couldn't understand what was going on, nor could we. What had happened to these two people who were so in love?

In part, the Jetsons happened. The Olive Pit happened. And every little question soon became an imposing and unyielding barometer of our entire relationship. All of these seemingly petty considerations transformed themselves into a body of evidence against the notion that we could overcome our differences and find a way to be happy together.

Parenthood was a stage we used to play out our own personal dramas with each other. We were battling each other for control of our household and our relationship. I'd really like to say it was all Layla's fault. And I suppose I can since I'm the one writing this book. So therefore:

IT WAS ALL LAYLA'S FAULT

That feels great. Unfortunately, it's just not true. Anyone can see that. Let me try something a bit closer to the truth:

IT WAS, ON BALANCE, MOSTLY LAYLA'S FAULT

There. That's comforting, and I like the way it points to how fair I am about things. I don't point fingers; I review the facts, and then come up with a balanced assessment (note the phrase "on balance").

But I'm really trying to be honest, so I suppose I should at least write the truth, which is this:

MARRIAGE IS A NO-FAULT ARRANGEMENT. LOVE MEANS NEVER HAVING TO SAY YOU'RE SORRY....

...and every other cliché that could someday haunt you when you're feeling alone and melancholy. There is no absolute truth. We both wanted different things out of our relationship —that's the closest I can come to it. I wanted us to spend more time together, and spend more time together as a couple. And I wanted Layla to want what I wanted.

To find out what Layla wanted, log on to her website at: www.michaelisaliarandfortherecordonbalancemostlyatfault butirefusetostooptohislevelandwriteabookaboutit.com

You may ask yourself, as I have too, doesn't something like cancer bring you together? Don't you just forget all the other shit and get back to the treasures that brought you to each other?

The answer is – of course you do. For about ten minutes. Just before the end credits roll and the movie ends. I know that's the cynical answer. What I believe to be true is that cancer, or childbirth, or a death in the family tends to exacerbate problems that already exist by – at the very least – providing new openings for them to jump out of.

Our break-up is not a big sloppy fighting-all-over-the-place type of mess. It's not the drop down drag out assault that my parents' divorce was. Hell it's not even a divorce yet, just a separation that begins in October. Maybe that's why it's so calm thus far. My separation is quiet and amicable and sad. Very sad. There have been so many times I've cried in the shower these past few months, not quite sure what the tears were about other than catharsis and some sort of shedding of a sadness I feel. My marriage certainly played its part. I don't think I'm much of a candidate for woe-is-me status though. We had several good years of marriage, we produced a great kid, and neither of us, I think, has become a psycho.

Several of my friends tell me that God never gives you more than you can handle. Not only does my atheism not accept such a notion, it's beginning to make me look like a genius. Ironically....I mean, I guess it's irony....I find my new apartment on September 12th because no one is apartment hunting that day except maybe other cancer survivors who also survived the collapse of the Twin Towers and are anxious to get on with surviving the end of their marriage. The girl who is subletting the apartment tells me she "thinks" she may have already sublet the place to someone two days ago, but she hasn't heard back from the girl and since there are thousands of people still unaccounted for in New York as of today, she doesn't know what it means that the girl hasn't called back. I have a very eerie sense about the whole thing, and I hate the idea of taking the apartment from someone who may have been lost or who lost someone in the tragedy 25 blocks away, but this is the first place I've seen that could work for me so I try my best to sell myself and hope that the other girl is alive, well, and no longer interested in the apartment. Two days later, with no further sign of the other girl, I'm given the keys to my new home.

Now comes the fun part. My wife and I decided not to tell anyone we were splitting up until I had a new place secured. Obviously, the first person we need to tell is our six-year-old son.

I remember when my parents took my older sister and me into their bedroom when I was seven years old and broke the news to us that my Dad had a new job and we were going to be moving from Huntington, New York to Minneapolis, Minnesota. Not only that, my mother was going to have a baby. What I remember most about this moment in my life is how I comforted myself with the thought that I was, unlike most kids from New York, a Minnesota Vikings football fan, and now I'd be closer to Fran Tarkenton (the former New York Giant) and the rest of the team. The news of a new brother or sister was more important to my sister. I thought it was, you know, kind of cool, but a minor development compared to going to Vikings games on a regular basis. In the end my father's job fell through, and we never moved to Minnesota, though I did have a little baby brother nine months later.

When I ask my friends for advice about how to speak to my son, some suggest I emphasize that he's actually "lucky to have two houses." I'm struck at how we try so hard to raise intelligent children, and then when it comes to emotional issues, some people think it's a good idea to treat them like idiots. "Hey son, your family is going to split apart and you're only six and don't really understand and you probably feel like you may never see your father again, or maybe you think he doesn't love you enough to want to live with you or worse you've heard about parents who divorce and fight and probably you feel that a lot of this is your fault but hey.....*you're lucky*....you get to have two houses!"

I suppose that means I'm lucky too. I get to have another piece of horrible news to break to my son. I did fine with the speech about my illness back in April. So I decide to treat this like what it is...a massive bummer that someday, hopefully, will turn out to be better for all of us. All day long I steel myself. I try to imagine how he will take the news and I keep repeating to myself: "He will be destroyed, so be prepared and try to comfort him." Just because kids can bounce back more quickly from adversity doesn't mean they don't hurt as much or more than we do.

I get home, look at Layla, and nod to her that this is the moment. My son, I'm thinking, is like me back in February when I suddenly got a call from Dr. Faust saying there was something on my lung. Life for him is good – difficult at times but overall fun and interesting.

Except I'm about to tell him something that will tear all of that apart and he has no idea that it is coming (Layla and I don't fight in front of him nor do we bad mouth each other and we're still moderately affectionate with each other). I was 40 when I got hit with my bad news. He's all of 6 and a half.

I tell him: "Luke. Mommy and I are going to separate. We're not going to live together anymore." In all my ordeal with illness, in all the difficult fights I've had with my wife, I have never felt the kind of pain I feel at this very moment. I can rationalize all I want, but in my soul I feel I'm inflicting the most horrible evil on the person I cherish the most in the world....the single most important reason I've been fighting so hard to conquer my cancer.....Luke. I see his brow start to wrinkle in slow motion and the tears start to form in his eyes. I'm surprised at how immediately he grasps the news and reacts like you'd expect....with tears and cries of "I don't want you to," and "Why Daddy? Why?"

His mother hugs him as hard as she can and tries to fight back her own tears. I try as best as I can to explain the situation. "Mommy and I are not happy living together. We don't want to do it anymore. We love you and will always be your Mommy and Daddy no matter what." And so on. I want so badly to distract him, or say something false and encouraging, but I fight the urge till the end.

He looks up at me in shock and says: "I don't want to talk about this anymore. I want to watch T.V." We say okay, and let him distract himself for a while. The Power Puff Girls are on, "saving the world before bedtime," and the three of us are doing whatever we can to get involved in their mission instead of thinking about what just transpired in our living room. Things have gone about as well as we could hope for, meaning dreadfully, but I am at least relieved that no matter what happens, I won't have to break this news again.

Enema Mine

Years ago, when men's marriages fell apart, they headed for the nearest bar to drink away their troubles. There is an intrinsic value in the numbing effect of alcohol. It allows a man to get his mind off what's gone wrong and to search for some sort of deeper truth within himself. I'm not much of a drinker and the deep truth within me is that I've simply got to get on with the choices I've made and try to build from there. So I do the next best thing. I go to IKEA.

I need a couch to sleep on in my new apartment. I select one and arrange for it to be delivered in a week. I buy a few pots and pans, a set of silverware, a table and a couple of shelves. What I really want to do is just move to IKEA altogether. I could work out of the Home Office section, eat my meals in the Restaurant, entertain in the Living Room area or play with my son in the Kids Room. Luke could grow up speaking Swedish and being really tolerant of others.

I know this sounds insane, but I am in need of some stability. Even our daily lives are beginning to resemble madness. Yesterday we received a letter from Luke's school, announcing that the New York City Police Department is fully cooperating with school staff to determine if the white-powdered envelope found on school property is anthrax. On top of that, I just found out that my friend Susan has breast cancer again. She'd been in remission for twelve years. I'm really thrown for a loop when I hear that after twelve years she's back dealing with the viper again. Her setback is a setback for all of us. I try to encourage her and offer my solidarity. I don't believe that Susan's misfortune is in any way an indicator of what will happen to me, but I'm starting to feel a strange buzzing inside, as if there were a tiny adrenaline leak somewhere in my brain. Maybe if IKEA won't take us, we can just pack up and move to Sweden.

The day before my furniture arrives, I head up to the Lymphoma Lounge, and dutifully submit to the tyranny of the CAT scan donut. Five days later, Portlock tells me there's a possible "abnormality" in my intestine.

There's something so matter of fact when she speaks to me.... it's not casual or flippant, just very very direct. She was described to me once as being "excellent clinically, though a bit cold", and even though part of me always wants my doctor to hold my hand and tell me to "hang in there" (that's what doctors usually say to cancer patients.... we patients say "good luck" to each other) I appreciate that she seems to be vested in finding out the truth and telling me what she thinks it means. Hell, somebody's got to do it and I guess we can be friends and hold hands when things turn out all right for me, if ever.

She says I need to have a fluoroscopy test to confirm the radiologist's suspicion about my CAT scan. A few days later Layla comes with me to the Arnold and Marie Schwarz Pavilion behind the hospital, on 67th street. I'm led into a new room with a new type of machine and I'm given a new beverage to drink before my new test. The nurse is a man named Jack, who is kind, funny, and likes to call himself my "valet." The machine is a fluoroscope which I'm later told will just keep beaming me with X-rays while the barium beverage courses its way through my system and lights up my insides.

Barium. You look at its white chalkiness and try in some way to convince yourself it's just a bad imitation of a milk shake. The same way the barium tea I have at all my CAT scans is just a bad version of iced tea. Luckily, years of beer guzzling in college taught me how to shut off my olfactory sensations and chortle down large quantities of liquid, so I'm able to disconnect my sense of smell and drink most of the barium in one gulp, and then the rest in another. It tastes like chalk, not that I've ever really tasted chalk before.

I lay down on the table and another doctor comes in. Asian. Female. I can't remember her name. She flips on the fluoroscope, and we watch the greenish monitor as it projects the pathways of my intestines. "What are we looking for?" I ask innocently. "This dark spot here," she says, in like two seconds, pointing at what looks like a broccoli floret with a dark spot on its stem.

Fuck. The broccoli-looking thing is what's called my small bowel (or small intestine), located just below my stomach, and the dark spot is another mass, which Portlock later christens "The Blob". Like the mass that preceded it in my lung, The Blob needs to be removed and/or destroyed. I hate the way the import of these discoveries sinks in; I'm laid out on a table, looking up at fluorescent lights, and through these strange technologies I'm looking into myself and seeing trouble. It's like waking up from a seemingly peaceful sleep and being told by your bedmate that you were screaming bloody murder all night. You can't believe it, and yet you feel…what is it? Guilty? Is that what this feeling is?

Soon Jack is in the room, showing me where to go to get dressed and just being one of the kindest human beings of all time. Thank you Jack's mother and father, wherever you are.

The doctor tells me on the way out to call if I have any trouble with my bowels because of the barium.

The next morning, I follow my normal urge to defecate but I detect a bit of constipation once I'm seated on the porcelain. "Must be the barium," I think. I've never taken any laxatives in my life, and Nanna Rose, my enema-enthusiast grandmother, has been dead for 30 years.

So it doesn't occur to me to try to help the process along, and since the doctor said to call if I had any trouble, and a bit of constipation certainly isn't "trouble", I just get up and go on with my day at the office.

Hours later, I still haven't voided, even though I've made one further attempt at doing so to no avail. I guess at this point I am officially constipated. The trouble really begins in the evening, around 9PM, when I make another ill-fated attempt to empty my bowels. It seems that no matter how hard I push, nothing will come out. Not only that, the muscles in my abdomen and rear end are starting to feel kind of sore. So I pop down to my local CVS pharmacy, buy some stool softener, gobble a couple of gel caps down, and think the matter dealt with. The instructions on the package promise a bowel movement sometime in the next six hours.

An hour later, I go back into the bathroom and push really hard, trying to just deploy the fucker out of me. But no dice. What's worse – this time my muscles seem to spasm, and the cramps are now really, really painful. I feel like my insides are gonna rip apart any second. I leave a message for Steven, who I know is on call, and he calls me right back and tells me to go back to the pharmacy and buy some glycerin suppositories. By now it's 10PM and the CVS is just about to close and I'm thinking....this better be it. I go back into the laxative section and buy the suppositories. When I go to pay, I try to imagine what's going through the mind of the checkout girl who'd just sold me the gel caps an hour ago. Whatever....I just can't help wondering. She's probably trained not to get too involved in people's problems, but I know she's seeing some rectal distress in my eyes or something.

I ram a suppository up the downside, and quickly feel the urge again so I give it my all. This time my muscles spasm so badly I can barely stand back up, and I'm caught somewhere between pushing and holding back....uncontrollably so. I pull my pants on, grab my cellphone and make a mad dash for the door. I'm trying to walk from my knees up, because taking a full step only seems to aggravate the pain.

CVS is closed. I head west in the direction of a Rite Aid which I'm praying is open 24/7, but I know that failing that I can go to St. Vincent's hospital another eight blocks on and they must have, I fantasize, some kind of machine that just sucks out whatever you've got stuck inside of you. Like when Richard Gere supposedly had that gerbil stuck up his sphincter....I know this is just an urban legend but I'm sure that every doctor's heard it by now and one of them must have thought to invent a machine like this....just in case it was ever REALLY needed. I hook up with Steven again on the phone. He tells me to relax, my insides only feel like they'll tear, but they won't. I trust Steven immensely, but I'm pretty sure...maybe it's the pain...that he's gonna be wrong at least once in his life and if this just happens to be that time, I'm completely fucked. I'm ready to burst. His instructions are to buy something called mineral oil. I get to Rite Aid and dash through its still open doors. As I head downstairs I realize that I didn't think to take my wallet on my way out. I grab madly through my pockets and find, miraculously, a five dollar bill. I pay and start to head back home, although at this point I'm really thinking I ought to head for St. Vincent's, even though Steven told me it'd be a miserable and painful experience (As opposed to what? The misery and pain I'm in now??). It feels like one of the biggest decisions of my life....if I get home and this mineral oil doesn't work, I'm gonna have to call an ambulance because there's no way, in this excruciating pain, that I'm going to be able to walk back the fifteen blocks to the hospital. No way.

I get only two blocks away and Steven calls me on the phone again. "I just fucking realized I should have told you to buy a Fleet enema as well," he says. Son of a bitch. Now I don't even know if I've got the strength to make it the two blocks back to Rite Aid and then another two to back where I am and then another EIGHT to my apartment, where, if both the mineral oil and an enema fail I am at risk of dying from a burst abdomen. That enema's only going to increase the steam boiler pressure I'm already feeling, and then it's do or die. I decide to go back to Rite Aid one last time, and no sooner do I do so and hang up then I remember that I've only got three dollars left. It's eight blocks to my wallet, ten blocks to the hospital, and two blocks to Rite Aid and the withering likelihood that a pre-packaged enema costs less than three bucks. All I can think is, "how did I get myself into a predicament where my very life seems to depend upon the price of an enema?" For all the bad things you hear about cancer – the operations, the chemotherapy, the radiation, the hair loss and on and on – you never in your wildest imagination think that you could die because some multinational has jacked up their profit margin on a device that you shove up your ass, and yet....given the right set of circumstances, it can happen. My fear is subordinate only to my discomfort as I renegotiate the stairs down to Rite Aid's basement. My vision feels like it's blurring, and I have trouble bending down because of the pain in my gut, but I spot the enema and its price tag. Two dollars and nineteen cents. It is nothing short of a godsend; in spite of my atheism, I see evidence of a Divinity in a truly unexpected place.

Now it's all about the walk back home. I am really frightened, despite what Steven's said, that I may not make it. I don't need to take a crap anymore, I need to give birth to it. Don't women die in childbirth all the time, even in America? How are they ever going to explain that one to my son, I wonder, as I turn off 6th Avenue onto Bleecker Street. "Sorry Luke. Your Dad died in rectal childbirth. We did everything we could for him."

The pain seems to let up for an instant. Maybe it's the motion. Maybe I've turned an intestinal corner, as it were. I make it up to my apartment, grab the enema, and put myself into the same supine position that I see pictured on the package. I don't even take my jacket off. It's a now or never thing and I haven't got time for any inefficient movement whatsoever.

I hang on for all I'm worth as the pressure builds up. I feel like I've got the go-ahead, and place myself on the toilet seat and start to push. But nothing comes out. I can feel my muscles tearing. I look at the plunger next to the toilet and think incoherently about how I can create some sort of suction. HOW CAN I CREATE SUCTION, GOD? I begin to fantasize madly that I can reach inside myself and find some sort of a handle on this coffee can and just rip it out of me, even if it's to be followed by a placenta, or sudden death from blood loss, or whatever lurks above the granite now lodged deep within my butt. I'm not pushing anymore; I'm just locked into this muscle spasm that feels like it wants to come tearing out of my stomach and onto the floor. *Must...eliminate...deadly...invader.......*

Miraculously, it's over in an instant. The huge mass suddenly separates itself from me like a two- stage Apollo rocket...its flaming core tailing behind it as it plummets into the oceanic latrine water below. My muscles slip back into relaxed mode and I instantly realize that I have never felt this good in my life about anything. Ever. Whatever happens to me from here on out I can deal with it. I am saved. I am truly truly happy in this moment. The fear and the pain are gone.

One Close Call Deserves Another

At the end of October my father and I head out to the neighborhood he grew up in, as part of a project I've decided to undertake with my parents. I'm going to bring them to the neighborhoods they grew up in, my father in Belle Harbor, Queens, and my mother in Flatbush, Brooklyn, and I'm going to film them talking about their childhoods. And about each other (the good years anyway) and about us when we were kids.

My Dad is first. He picks me up at 7AM. Like everyone else in my family, he is a talker, and my only real concern is if I'll have enough battery power to keep up with his reminiscences. He talks as he drives. Tells me how he never really got along with his father. How his mother was the center of his life. How she was the only one he could really talk to. "My father wasn't a bad guy. I just couldn't ever get any good advice from him," he says.

I learn that my father's career, which began as a buyer for a department store (Abraham & Strauss), is a result of his having worked in my uncle's mattress factory in Pomona, California for a summer. One day my father emerged from his work covered in feathers and glue and beheld a man in a suit and tie who was chatting with my uncle. My father asked what the man did for a living and he said: "I'm a buyer for a department store." My father decided right then and there that he wanted to wear what that guy wore – a suit and tie – and so when he returned to Rockaway, he signed up for the A&S buyer training program.

We reach his house on Beach 131st Street, so named because it's part of a series of streets that end at the sand of Rockaway Beach.

He stands proudly in front of his boyhood home and proclaims, "This is it. This is my house." He points to a wall down the road, at the corner of Beach 131st and Newport Avenue. "You see that wall," he says. "Me and my best friend Pinky Goldner used to sit on that wall at night and talk about our lives growing up."

My intuition tells me to bring him to the wall, which I do. It's a white wall only about two feet off the ground. I sit him down and film for almost half an hour. We pack up and go home.

Sixteen days later, the fuselage of American Airlines flight 587 goes slamming into that very same wall. We watch the tape of the interview, my father and I, and notice that at one point we'd stopped the interview because of the noise of a plane flying overhead. A noise so loud that it was obvious to both of us that, given a difference of 16 days, we would never have had time to get out of the way.

I'm alive. Many others are dead. The fuselage could care less. And while I'm happy to have dodged another plane, so to speak, life is beginning to feel like a torrent of potshots aimed in my general direction.

I'm angry about having cancer again. Borderline furious. What happened to "thinking about this disease in terms of decades?" Where did "normal lifespan" go? How did I wind up getting sucked down the cancer vortex after only six months?

Portlock has sent me to a new surgeon, Dr. Martin Karpeh, even though I was hoping Dr. Rusch could operate on me again. But my new growth is a few inches south of her area of expertise, a distinction Nanna Rose would appreciate, I'm sure.

Karpeh is an abdominal surgeon. His voice is soft, the palms of his hands are as pillowy as sofa cushions, and his smile is warm and disarming. You look at him and you think: gentle, reassuring, caring. But at the same time, there's a confident, controlled measure to his bearing that speaks of precision and thoughtfulness, which are two not-bad-at-all characteristics when it comes to the guy who's going to operate on you. However, to my pleasant surprise he tells me at our first meeting: "Michael, don't get me wrong. I'd love to operate on you. It's what I do. But I have a non-surgical approach I want to try first." A non-surgical approach? I'm not sure if this is the number one greatest thing a surgeon could ever say to me, but it's got to be in the top two. My eyes light up with intrigue.

"MALT lymphomas in the stomach are sometimes treatable with antibiotics. Although yours appears to be in the area between the stomach and the small intestine, I recently read about a study in which a protocol of antibiotics worked for an abnormality like yours; that is, outside of the stomach. Of course I want Doctor Portlock to agree as well before I give you the go ahead."

I'm elated, but it is short-lived as a few hours later Portlock characterizes the probability of success as "close to unheard of." Nonetheless, she gives me her blessing to try it. Even if it doesn't work, my new blob is unlikely to grow much in the interim. Thanks Blob. Or whatever you are. Indeed whatever it is, I'm told, will not be confirmed until I have a biopsy done. And since we need to be sure it is what the doctors think it is, namely, the bastard cousin of my last lymphoma, I am sent to none other than Colonel...I mean Doctor... Kurtz to try to biopsy it. Another great name from literature destined to send a probe down my throat.

Unfortunately the blob is at the exact geographic midpoint of my body: too far down the top of me to get with a normal probe, and too far up my bottom to reach with anything short of medieval. Kurtz selects a 42-inch pediatric endoscope, the kind of implement that could probably reach your inner child, if called upon. He knocks me out…out cold… with Demerol. It kind of ticks me off because I don't get to enjoy the Demerol buzz, although I'm fast coming to the conclusion that being unconscious has been highly underrated in my life.

And how right I am. I wake up to learn that 42 inches just wasn't long enough for Kurtz to reach the Blob. He warned me this might occur, but I am still miserable at having undergone this whole rigmarole for nothing. The Blob is either a slow growing MALT lymphoma like I had last time, or a fast growing new type of lymphoma, or else something called a soft tissue sarcoma. Either way, its lease is up in the next 4-6 weeks or so, unless the program of antibiotics works some kind of magic.

Just as the medical details are unclear, my state of mind is…frankly….a bit in flux as well. The rest of my life isn't quite shining in glory, unless you compare me to a war refugee from the Sudan, in which case I apologize for taking all my blessings for granted. But I'm suffering mentally, and as my sage-though-cocaine-addicted college roommate used to say to me, in his inimitable Country-Boy-From-Tennessee way: "Mahk. You caynt equate sacalogical payn and physical payn. Thur two different animals."

It looks like I'll live….literally…..which is a start. And I really like Karpeh. He's the first African-American doctor I've come across in all this time, which makes me think that he must have really been at the top of his class to make it this far. Later I reflect on this theory and decide that, actually, the world would be an enormously better place if white people like me stopped making *any* assumptions about people based on their race. I had the same must-have-been-magna-cum-laude assumptions about my other surgeon, Doctor Rusch, because she is a woman, so I'm going to try to extend my non-assumption making to include people of other genders as well. It's just that, as my Aunt Blanche told me years ago, a drowning man will clutch at anything he can, and I'm hunting for any reason at all to believe in my surgeons. It's to the point where, if Doctor Karpeh were to tell me he'd won, say, a lacrosse tournament when he was younger, I'd find a way to interpret that as: "Well, there's a clear indication that he has excellent eye-hand coordination, a fundamental skill in abdominal surgery." I call Dr. Faust to see if he knows Karpeh from around the Gastro-Enterology Circuit and he says: "I don't know him. But I'm sure you're in excellent hands. They've got a pretty rigorous screening process up at Memorial Hospital."

In other words moron, calm the fuck down.

Department Of Cash

Did I mention that I'm going broke? It's a special kind of broke – one that you don't hear about too often. I call it "rich broke." Some people who suffer from rich broke will try to get you to feel sorry for them. Not me. If I did, I'd have to also try to get you to feel sorry for me because I got cancer. Frankly, I just don't have that kind of time, and I'm not deserving of pity either. But cancer and bankruptcy are indeed interesting bedfellows.

Here's what happens when you get rich broke. You start out rich, or in my case, as a man of means. You've got your steady income, in my case derived from a production company I own that makes TV commercials for European TV. It's a lucrative business, even though it's probably contributing to the ruin of European culture. Advertising has a way of doing that. You own a fancy apartment (where your former wife now lives), which we do because we got lucky enough to buy it at the ebb of the real estate market in the early nineteen nineties, just before our neighborhood became desirable to live in for people who either didn't deal crack, or who'd gotten rich on the crack epidemic and wanted to settle down. These days when an apartment in the building goes up for sale, models and movie stars show up to bid on it. In some ways it makes you feel small – as if you've made the neighborhood safe for models and movie stars, and now you should graciously accept their pay off and move to a neighborhood devoid of models and movie stars. They're so grateful for your contribution that they will pay more than your asking price, and in some cases, even forego moving in at all. When you're a model or movie star, sometimes owning "just for show" is enough.

So anyway, you've got your money mojo working just great, you're gainfully employed, you're comfortably housed, you've even got your no-budget documentary film (about Melvin Van Peebles, the filmmaker and maverick) going on with your friend Joe, that you shoot whenever you have a free weekend and that may some day bring you artistic acclaim – and then you find out you have cancer. Or rather, you enter the world of cancer, which means you need to see dozens of doctors before you even know what the hell's going on; then, once they think they've figured out what *is* going on, they promote you to Cancer Treatment World. Much to your chagrin, though, all of this cancer tourism takes time, and these are not the kind of appointments that you can generally schedule for after work, or during your lunch hour.

I tell Joe about my cancer – a disease he lost his mother to – and he is as supportive and empathic as a friend can possibly be. He's all: "Don't *even* worry about the movie. Just focus on getting better." While a really magnificent guy, Joe is possessed of the same type of warped mind as I, which may be leading him to wonder, just as I do, if our movie is going to someday wind up being in memory of me. In any case, neither of us is saying so.

Over at my day job, I've got a few things going for me. First of all, I own my company, so I don't have to ask anyone for time off to go see my doctors. I'm also able to come home from my appointments and cry if I feel the urge, which I often do, instead of returning to the office. I have people in my office who can lie and say that I'm "in a meeting" or "on a conference call" when really I'm talking to my doctor on the phone and learning about some new horror or indignity. That's the good part.

The bad part is, it's *my* ass at work. With all due respect to the wonderful women I work with, I'm the guy responsible for bringing in and mollifying our clients. I also have to make sure there's enough dough in the bank to pay everyone. And I've got to figure out just how much I'm going to tell our clients about my illness, and when. This is even more awkward than telling my friends, because my friends don't think about the economic impact of my illness (with one notable exception…when I tell my oldest friend Gary about my illness – he being someone I've known since I was a boy of three – he falls silent before explaining to me in his gentlest voice that he is "just trying to figure out if you owe me any money"). I am really concerned that my clients might see me as someone bearing the mark of Cain – tainted, and in some weird way even contagious. This is irrational of course, but that's the way people often think. I handle this dilemma by having Elena and Stephanie do the "he's in a meeting" charade for the first couple of months as in:

"He'd love to chat, but he's in a meeting."

"I'll have him call you when the meeting's over."

"I'm pretty sure he sent the check, but I can't ask him right now. He's in a meeting."

Once I've got my diagnosis and know when and where I'm having my surgery, I'm no longer in a meeting. I call my clients up and let them know that I'll be away from work for about a month. I tell them I have cancer, but I'm going to be all right.

"Tengo un cancer, pero' todo va a estar bien."

"Ho un cancro. Ma non c'e' da preoccuparsi."

"J'ai une maladie qui s'appelle 'lymphome', mais ce n'est pas grave."

They are universally stunned, and kind, and generous, and encouraging. Maybe something got lost in the translation – are people really this beautiful? They tell me "don't worry, we'll work with your people until you get better." It's great really – I am so moved by their kindness and understanding. I continue to believe that even though I've gotten shafted in terms of Overall Luck, I have been really lucky when it counted most.

The only nagging problem I have is that someone forgot to tell my lymphoma not to come back. Believe me – it's more than a minor oversight. A one-time health crisis is fairly commonplace in the world of business; executives are constantly taking paid leave to have pacemakers installed, or heart valves stented, or to chew the fat over at the local Betty Ford clinic. But doing it two times means, "we have no way of knowing when this may happen again." Two times means, "maybe the guy's gonna die." Two times is fuckin' pushing it.

Everybody's still nice, but like me, they're a bit on the pissed off side about the recurrence. I'd sold them the prognosis my doctors sold me. The bit about thinking of my disease in terms of decades. Further complicating matters is the economic picture at large. The economy sucks. The advertising business is in freefall. The dollar's been strong all year, which makes services like the ones my company provides artificially expensive for my clients. And no one wants to come film in New York either, not after the Trade Center gets attacked and some anthrax-wielding nut is on the lam.

The final tally for me is a seventy percent drop off in revenue. Does my having cancer have anything to do with my business going south? Who knows? I'm sure it doesn't help.

All I know is, the whole thing has left me a bit short on cash. But I'm rich broke, which means I still have enough to eat, and support my child. My parents have helped me out. My health insurance covered most of my medical expenses. So I'm not desperate and starving. I'm just too poor to continue living in the manner to which I have become accustomed. That's what rich broke is – a more impoverished version of yourself. You order a cheaper bottle of wine in a restaurant. You panic at the soon-to-arrive tuition bill for your kid's school. You buy seltzer instead of Perrier, generic instead of brand name, quantity instead of quality. Everything looks fine, but something is clearly wrong.

That is what's really scary about rich broke – it's far less overt than say, being a bag lady. The pain you feel is more psychological than physical. You're not hungry; you're humiliated. You're also dangerous to yourself and others. Poor people are, for the most part, docile. It's sad, but true. Humiliated people are crazy. They take up crimes like embezzlement. They lead secret lives as male prostitutes. They kill themselves and their families in the heat of the moment.

One other telltale characteristic of the rich broke is that we have copious amounts of frequent flyer miles. I'm talking in the six and seven digits. In my case, I accumulated all my miles back when I was a big shot. I got miles for all my business trips; double miles for flying business class, triple miles for first class. I got one of those credit cards that award you a mile for each dollar you spend. I charged everything I could, from pencils to wardrobe to gigantic film lights. Did I pick up the tab at our business lunch, you ask, just because I wanted the miles? Of course not. I mean, yes. I mean, not to the best of my recollection, your Honor.

I decide to use my miles to fly the coop for a week. Although I don't expect to die even if I have to have another operation, I'm not taking any chances. I've been living in the moment for a long while now, and I'm probably not going to be able to travel again until winter. I want to see some of my friends and I can't wait around for a larger slot of time to take advantage of.

I take off on Delta Airlines, First Class (80,000 miles). Destination Rome. Reserving a seat on the airplane using my mileage – a task normally about as simple as finding tofu in a steakhouse – is ridiculously easy this time. Everyone is still afraid to fly, and I suppose I might be too if I didn't have a malignant tumor in my intestine. Perspective is a beautiful thing sometimes.

Two seats in front of me I see the actor Henry Winkler, as in, the Fonz. Every third passenger on the plane walks by him and gives him the Oh-My-God-It's-Fonzie-But-I-Musn't-Let-On-That-I'm-Looking look. I am fortunate to have boarded before Mr. Fonzarelli, so I am spared this ritual that I find so uncomfortable. I'm like everyone else around famous people. I get that weird adrenaline burst and feel my cheeks get flush. When a celebrity is around, it seems like you've got the choice of either acknowledging them in that awkward and friendly way, like using the old stock phrase: "I'm a big fan of your work" even though you've seen maybe one-twentieth of the things they've done, or else you can make believe you don't see and/or recognize them at all. You pretend you've developed this sudden and intense fascination with the spot just above their head, or just past their ear. In your mind you think "I'm cool because I'm not staring at Fonzie. I mean, Henry Winkler. Ordinary citizen."

Anyway, here I am on the plane, which is about half empty at take-off time. We're served a seafood platter appetizer with capers and lemon and – get this – a plastic knife to cut it with. My first thought is that this is just a hijacking deterrent, until I see that we've also been given a remarkably sharp metal fork. Sharp as in: "Ow that fucking hurts" sharp. I'm no expert on air piracy, but I don't see how a fork is that much less dangerous than a butter knife. But I guess people are jittery and symbolic actions are important even if they're not very well thought out.

I'm met at Rome airport by my friend Guido. Guido used to live in New York, back when he was known as Guido Go Ahead Laugh At My Name. Like most of the lasting relationships in my life, ours began with a high degree of mutual dislike bordering on enmity. He was a neurotic prick, and I was the same perfect non-judgmental human being I am today. I liked Guido's girlfriend Gina, which made him dislike me even more, even though I only liked her as in "like." One day Guido needed someone who could speak Italian to take over his job with the Torino Film Festival because he was going to be shooting his first feature film in the California desert. A story about the Manson family. The guy comes to this country and all he can think to do is a story about our slimiest citizen. Thanks Guido.

I take the job and he goes off to scout his movie. Six weeks later, he is back in New York because the financing of his masterpiece has completely fallen through. Now that we've got this film festival thing going on, we're suddenly spending a lot of time talking to each other. Then Gina takes off on vacation for the summer, Layla takes off to Beirut to finish her doctorate, and every night of the week Guido and I are at a bar on 2nd Street and Avenue A, drinking gin and tonics and talking about politics and women. We begin to form a bond.

Today, fifteen years later, we are like brothers. Guido is married to Nicoletta and they've got a couple of sweet little daughters that have rendered them reasonably content and woefully exhausted. I hang out with them and our friends Laura and Gherardo. We eat non-stop and talk about the World Trade Center, cancer, divorce, and Laura's recent nervous breakdown. I could write a book about my trip so far called "Europe on Five Valium a Day." At least the food is stunningly delicious.

I go to Paris for three days and hang out with Jean-Pierre and Julie. They are rich broke like me. We spend the night at Julie's chateau outside of Paris, which is, basically, an actual Chateau made up of about eighty rooms and several hundred acres. I'm given my own bedroom, bathroom and lounge. I'm thinking, "I'm getting divorced,

I have cancer, and I'm living the life of Louis the Fourteenth. There is an almost divine symmetry in this madness."

From Paris I go to Madrid for one day to meet with some of my clients. We have lunch with an ad agency guy who we suspect is a pedophile and we eat chorizo and discuss an upcoming project that we are pretty sure will never happen. This is pretty much standard operating procedure for the ad world. Pedophiles and upcoming projects that never happen. The chorizo is, instead, a welcome change to the routine.

No one is quite sure how to say goodbye to me. I try to explain that this time, even *I* don't think I'm going to the gallows, but it is little consolation to my friends. They know the reason I'm leaving in such a hurry is that I have a CAT scan the day after I get back, December 14th, to see if the antibiotics worked any magic. I'm just pleased to have seen my friends, and to have lived like a French king for a night.

First Man On Mars

Back home Luke is adjusting to our separation about as well as we could possibly hope. He says to me that he's no longer afraid because "I like your place and I like Mom's place." This is an enormous turning point for us. I wound up making a really good decision about my new apartment – just a lucky guess really – by taking one of the rooms and turning it into my son's bedroom. I sensed that if he had his own room he might start to feel like it was a home too. I sleep in the living room on a fold-out couch. My place is a one-bedroom railroad flat in the middle of the West Village that looks like a model plane enthusiast built it. Model as in "scale model." New York is full of these places where you're so grateful to raise your arms and not hit the ceiling that you don't mind how Lilliputian the rest of the apartment is. I know that size doesn't matter in sex, so I try to pretend that it doesn't matter in apartments either. And in a sense, it's true; no matter how small your penis, you still need a decent sized apartment.

One of the women who lives in my building tells me that her father was the man who built this place, that she herself has been here for thirty six years, and – she's sure I'd like to know – her uncle died in my very apartment years ago. I thank her for the history and decide then and there not to talk to anyone in my hallway ever again. Just in case anyone else's uncle died here.

I go for my umpteenth CAT scan the day after I return and try to visualize a shrunken tumor in my intestine. It is desperately trying to cling to the wall of my bowel, but it's being overwhelmed by a snowstorm of antibiotic particles, which blanket and smother it in an intense nuclear winter. It screams: "Help! I am a powerless tumor being overrun by modern drugs!" and it's got that comic book voice, going: "Can't....hold.....on....much...long...er..."

Four days later, I get the results. The Blob is still The Blob: unshrunken, unmoved, and unimpressed with the wonders of modern pharmacology. Not only that, it now appears that I've had The Blob with me since at least last February, when this whole odyssey began. The trouble with the imaging of a CAT scan is that when it looks at the bowel, which is where my blob lives and works, it has to snap a picture of any abnormality at the exact moment that the contrast dye injected into me is in that particular area. It's kind of like the way a camera at night can only capture the area lit by the flashbulb. Add to that the fact that the bowel is constantly moving itself. One thing I can say I've learned from my disease is this: Kodak will not save your life. Only living your life to its fullest will.

Portlock recommends I have The Blob removed surgically, and a week later I see Karpeh to schedule the operation. My antibiotic miracle was only an illusion, though I probably won't need chemo. I'm told it is highly unlikely that what I have in my intestine is an aggressive type of cancer that would need chemotherapy. Although recurrence is likely, it is also possible that it will never recur again. How long will I have to deal with this? Forever and perhaps never again. Monitoring is now a part of my life.

Karpeh sets me up for surgery on January 8th. At this time a scant year ago, I was planning a trip to Washington D.C. to protest the inauguration of George W. Bush. I was angry that the Supreme Court had halted the counting of ballots and, in essence, chosen who would be the next President. I walked around the capitol in the pouring rain holding a sign that said: "Hey Scalia. Pick Me." As usual, my impact upon world affairs was totally negligible, but I felt good for trying.

This year I'll be treated to a 5-7 day stay in the hospital. Unlike my last operation, I'll have to prove that everything's working by passing gas through my repaired intestine before I can get out of the hospital. In short, you cut the cheese, they cut you loose. Later I tell Luke about my operation and as expected, he likes the part about the farting.

Physically, other than the lymphoma, I'm doing great. I'm a God-like specimen, insofar as a short Jewish guy approaching age 42 can be considered God-like. Psychologically it's a tougher call. I'm struggling. I spend a lot of time reminding myself that I have a wonderful child. Spectacular child. A healthy and intelligent child. I have a sense of humor that in spite of everything (like for example, that it is often misguided and unfunny) is something that I can fall back on and always seem to find some reason to giggle. I have a family that loves me, supports me, even drives me nuts at times which is perhaps the best way to know that they are sincere. I have friends that I wouldn't swap for anyone else's and whose value I can honestly say I understand and appreciate deeply, as in, Marianas Trench deep. I'm still learning about the world I inhabit, still wonder at it most of the time, still feel like I haven't yet lost my shot at being the first man on Mars, a prediction of my childhood babysitter Mrs. Peterman.

One issue I still need to resolve is this: every time I have a doctor's appointment, my friends and family, who I've been keeping well-informed of my progress, start to call me. That would be okay if they called me, say, after I'd actually seen my doctor, but instead everyone's anxiety starts early in the morning, and so I'm finding that by 10AM of any appointment day, I've already fielded at least 6 phone calls. They go like this:

Friend: Hi Mike. I'm just calling to check in.

Me: Hi. You mean check in about my health?

Friend:	Yeah. Any news?
Me:	My appointment's not till this afternoon.
Friend:	Yeah I know.
Me:	So that would sort of preclude the news department until then.
Friend:	Yeah you're right. Well I'm sure everything's going to be fine.

Not only am I not making this conversation up, I've had it many, many times. I'm generally anxious on appointment days, and it's getting to be too much trying to deal with everyone else's anxiety, especially when there's nothing I can do anyway. It's a familiar type of love to a Jewish boy like me. It's called smothering. Luckily I'm able to solve this problem rather easily. I offer to e-mail everyone all the gory details of my life in exchange for not calling me on appointment days. They accept, only soon I am surprised to learn that some of my friends have begun to forward my e-mails to their friends, and they in turn are writing directly back to *me*. I start getting e-mail messages from people I've never met, offering support and solidarity.

The e-mail idea is an enormous relief from having to notify everyone individually, plus I begin to draw sustenance from my newfound audience of strangers. If this is what a revelation is, then I'll take every one I can get.

Survivor: Upper Eastside

I'm not asking for the moon, I'm just asking for a little break. There is no need for a chest tube for my intestinal operation. Nor is a spinal tap required. I assume that the Foley catheter is *de riguer* and try to console myself with the notion that somehow having experienced a Foley it will now be less unpleasant.

Me: (to myself): Yes it's a tube in your penis, but it's only temporary.

Myself (to me): I will defend my penis to the death.

I take my penis seriously, even if no one else does. It has been a losing battle thus far, and a battle that I might still be fighting today, except that just in the nick of time – a week before my operation to be exact – a nurse in my surgeon's office casually mentions to me that when I awaken there will be....get this.... a drainage tube jutting out from my nose.

My nose? Did anyone else see that kid on TV who could put a string through his nose and pull it out of his mouth? Is there a single person in this world, man or woman, black or white, rich or poor, sick or healthy, who can imagine a tube going up from his stomach and out through his nose and not cringe and cower and shake?

I can't. I wish I could muster a great display of heroism, or maturity, but the truth is I shudder to think of such a device. Is this the best system the great medical minds could come up with to drain excess fluid? Am I now to be led around by my nose?

This is truly bad. My friends ask me how I'm doing, I tell them I'm psyched up for the operation, which is true, and yet what I don't say is that all I'm thinking about is the nose tube. Everyone is asking me about coming to visit in the hospital and I sort of hem and haw because I fear my friends are just like me and the site of a tube hanging out my proboscis will be very slow in fading from memory. I try to persuade myself that this is just vanity, and since I know how ridiculous vanity is, I should really just try to forget about it. But I know there's something else to it. I'm afraid of the uneasiness, the avoidance of the whole thing in conversation when in all likelihood I'll be talking about how good I'm feeling and my friends will be saying how good I'm looking and neither of us will give voice to the presence of the long and rubbery probe coursing from my gut to my drainage tube via my schnoz. The same way that I sometimes desperately find myself trying not to stare at a woman's décolleté. At least in that case you can just look up, or try to frame your vision so it goes no lower than her neck. Plus, worst comes to worst, you fail in your mission and you're left with this mental picture of a fetching woman's bust. Not so with nose tubes. The only way not to see one is to close your eyes.

So I lie and say: "I'm not really sure how up for visitors I'll be." Or I say: "Hopefully I'll be out of the hospital so quickly again that you won't even have time to come see me." Or I say: "I'm not sure if I'll even get a private room. So it's hard to plan for visitors." For an instant I consider just being honest and saying: "I don't want you to see me with a nose tube hanging out of me", but I know that that'll just *create* an image in the mind of the would-be visitor that's sure to be even worse than the real thing.

A week before my surgery, I get a call from Karpeh's office saying that my operation is going to be postponed for a week because Karpeh has to do jury duty. Part of me is understanding and civic minded. Another part of me is thinking: "Whoever the guy is, whatever the crime, he's guilty. Now give me back my surgeon." I just want to get this over with.

I'm prepared to stay in the hospital longer this time because even if I have a truly speedy recovery, they won't let me out unless I can prove that I can eat and fully digest my food. Since they have to wait at least a day or two to even feed me, there's no way I'll be out in one day like last time. But still, I don't want to stay a minute longer than necessary.

At last the day arrives. I check in at the hospital, head up to pre-op, and don my beloved gown and cap.

However, this operation is different from the get-go. Instead of being wheeled into the operating room on a gurney, in a state of near total sedation, this time I am just wheeled in by wheelchair and hooked up to the anesthesia once I get to the O.R.. I flick on some music I've brought along, a "Crystal Blue Persuasion" cover by Morcheeba, and I'm on my way. We enter the O.R. and the nurse there politely asks me to please climb up on the table and lay down. The operating table is covered in bright green sheets, and honestly, laying yourself down upon it is just not as simple as hopping up onto any other surface in the world. I mean, try asking a cow to hop up onto a butcher's table. Sure, he may do it willingly if he's flying on morphine, or whatever it is they sedate cows with, but try asking him when he's listening to "Crystal Blue Persuasion" and just starting to relax a bit. I have little choice but to comply.

Now that I'm single and available and have a decent rap worked out to explain the shower cap ("I'm just holding it for a friend"), there is of course no sign of the Indian beauty from last time. Just my luck.

The first person to introduce herself is my anesthesiologist. She starts me on a mild sedative as track two ends (U2's "One"....

it has that ethereal guitar riff and it plays like a smooth intro into the netherworld) and track 3, Dylan's "Most of the Time", begins to sneak through my brain wires. Several people dressed in a green color matching my sheets pull on masks and begin wheeling various machinery towards me. You know that beep...beep...beep you always hear on TV during operations? It is torn straight from the pages of reality. I think it may be the heart monitor but I'm just guessing. I lay there for a few minutes waiting for my surgeon to come in and thinking about what a total state of surrender I am entering. Has everyone in the room had a good night's sleep? Anybody fought with his or her spouse this morning? If so, is there anything I can do to help? I guess this is what happens when you're an atheist like me.... right at the time you should be thanking the Almighty, or repenting for your sins, you absurdly search for any last thing that might make a difference. I hear applause, but it's only the live recording of Dave Matthews covering the Beatles song "In My Life", a.k.a. track 4.

Karpeh walks in. I ask him the question that's been burning in my mind for a week. "How'd it go at Jury Duty?" He says: "I got out of it. But it's my fifth postponement, so I don't know how much longer I can hold them off." I know what he's talking about. In New York City the system allows you to postpone 3 times by mail, but every subsequent postponement requires an appearance in person down at 60 Centre Street. I myself was down there just a month ago on my fourth postponement. They still had no phone service there because it got knocked out when the Twin Towers went down, but anyway, I digress. That belongs in the episode known as SURVIVOR: FINANCIAL DISTRICT which aired during fall season.

He asks me what I'm listening to and it just happens to be at this very moment Miles Davis' "Kind of Blue" (a suggestion of my friend Rob Stewart, poet and music aficionado). My surgeon, it turns out, is a big Miles fan, as is his chief resident, who is standing on the other side of the table just near my head. We start going on about Miles, have you read the Quincy Troupe biography, etcetera etcera and all of a sudden I'm thinking things are kind of looking up. We've got some harmonic convergence going on here. They slip a mask over my face, tell me to start breathing deeply and there I go.....fade to black.

A couple hours later I wake up in the recovery room. My first thought is "I do not have a tube sticking out of my nose." No one is around my bed, but it feels like only seconds before I realize that my nose is just like it always has been. Unencumbered, untethered, unmistakably free! Not only that, I haven't got anything artificial protruding from the land of Dick! Nor have I got a spinal tap in me, even though I thought Karpeh had said I was to get one. But no, it's just me, my nose, my dick, and my newly modified intestines. I'm so relieved because I know that these are all good signs. Soon I see my brother Andrew and Layla walk into the recovery room, followed by my mother and father. I can sense from their expressions that the operation was a success. A few hours later, I am wheeled up to the 15th floor and into my room.

I try to get up and walk around the ward almost immediately, because I remember that this walking sped my recovery a great deal last time. I actually manage to do one lap, pushing my I.V. pole around in front of me at an average speed of 0.0003 miles per hour. Good sense then dictates that getting back into bed might not be the worst of ideas. I haven't had anything to eat or drink all day, nor will I get anything until two days from now, so a lot of my thought process is taken up by a recurrent desire to drink something. Anything. I can speak clearly for about twenty seconds, after which my voice begins to sound like I am gargling marbles. Every ten minutes my morphine drip pipes in another .01 milligrams, and I have the option to squeeze a button and get a double dose at the same ten-minute interval. They quickly become the longest ten-minute intervals of my life.

Everyone goes home around 6PM and shortly thereafter a nurse comes in and informs me that if I don't urinate in the next two hours they'll have to give me a Foley catheter. Talk about motivation. I had a Foley inserted during my last surgery, but at least I was under general anesthesia at the time. Here they're gonna do it battlefield style. I protest that I haven't had anything to drink, but she says it doesn't matter because I've been receiving fluids through my I.V.. I say to the nurse: "Get me out of this bed." I stand up and try to relocate the muscles connected to my bladder. To my great dismay, I seem to have no muscular memory at all. Anesthesia causes the bladder to spasm, but mine seems to be playing a game of hide and seek. The nurse turns on the faucet in my bathroom and I try to focus on the sound of the running water. Talk about pressure. "Here bladder bladder. Here bladder bladder. Come out come out wherever you are." I try to visualize great pees of the past. The Philippe Stark-designed urinals in a Paris cafe. The first one of the morning into the Colorado River on my Grand Canyon expedition. I channel rain, and waterfalls, and clouds bursting at the seams. Mercifully, after a few moments, I feel a tiny droplet wending its way out, like a desperate hiker struggling to pull himself up a steep mountainside (alright, maybe not that steep). Seconds later the floodgates open and I am home free. Phew!

I don't get much sleep the first night; ten or fifteen minutes every hour, but that's it. By 5:30 I'm up and pushing myself and my I.V. pole around the ward again. Slowly but steadily, the other inmates arise and make their way out to the hallway, which runs all the way around the rectangular floor. The protocol seems to be to smile politely at people as you pass them, a sort of clearly-this-sucks-have-a-nice-day kind of smile. Cancer isn't at all particular about who it strikes, and this being New York, you see all types. For some reason, I guess it must be the season, I have Martin Luther King's "I Have A Dream" speech in my head, the part where he says "Black men and white men, Jews and Gentiles...." and so on. Once again there appear to be a lot of Russians on my floor, with names like Yelena and Nadya, though there is a Bree (I guess upper East Side socialite), a Norman, and a woman named Rose Wong.

It's a weird place to meet people....even though you're all wearing the same version of the standard-issue schmatta/robe/gown, it feels like you're meeting each other while naked. Everyone...literally everyone... is hooked up to some sort of I.V., has some sort of tube or something sticking out of them (places like their nose, or their chest, or their stomach), and nearly everyone's blood and/or urine is on display (I am fortunately spared this particular indignity this time, but it is really just a matter of luck).

You can see into everyone's room as you pass. Loss of privacy is a given in the hospital, what with all the updates to your I.V., the temperature taking, the blood pressure checking. Also a lot of people have special "conditions" such as an allergy to latex or an intense sensitivity to infection. I know this because their rooms have giant signs saying: "LATEX ALLERGY" or "REVERSE PRECAUTIONS - MUST WEAR MASK". I can only imagine how terrific it makes them feel to have their weaknesses advertised on billboards like this, although in all fairness, there is an extraordinary amount of care put in at Memorial Hospital to respect what little dignity a patient is left with. You sort of have to tell yourself: "Hey man it's a cancer ward. Suck it up." I do about fifteen laps (just over a mile) then get back to my room and do twenty-five sit-ups (just kidding). I've unthinkingly brought the book "Kitchen Confidential" to read during my stay, which is a non-stop description of many of the world's great foods. Duck a' l'Orange. Pesto-infused mashed potatoes. Steak frites and swordfish tartare. I don't think I'm a masochist, I think I'm just an idiot. Here I am starving to death and I'm reading the literary equivalent of the Food Channel.

Visiting hours, given my family and friends, are pretty hilarious at times. Highlights include Kasino, my Mom and my brother showing each other what they learned in yoga (I huddle in the remaining 14 centimetres of my room and watch), Layla falling asleep in my bed for two hours while I am relegated to a nearby chair (other than that, she's been an absolute doll this go-round. Maybe now that the pressure of our marriage is off, we can return to a richer kindness toward each other), my father nodding off on a bi-minute basis thanks to the pain killers he's taking for his broken shoulder, and a seemingly endless discussion among visitors about cellphone plans and reliability (what is this world coming to?). I do my best to answer the questions "how do you feel?" and "have you farted yet?" and "who was that Spanish-speaking patient I got connected to when I tried to call your room?" (Answer: I have no idea, except apparently this person kept telling everyone "Michael esta en su casa").

By day three they put me on a liquid diet, thanks to my having passed some bona fide wind. Next thing I know a person wearing a waiter's outfit comes to my room and hands me something called a Room Service Menu. Under appetizers it has Jello: orange, cherry, or grape. Entrees are consommé: beef or chicken. But after three days with no food or drink, I feel as if I'm at the Hotel du Cap in Antibes. I can't believe how civilized the whole process is. Instead of them bringing you a tray of whatever they choose at whatever time they choose, whether you're hungry or not, you just dial 2200 on your phone and within fifteen minutes or so your order arrives.

The next day, I switch to the soft food diet (complete with new menu), and I am eating pretty well. Only still no bowel movement, the holy grail of post-abdominal surgery. By day four, I am practically jogging around the ward, having no trouble getting any food down (I eat fish, and rice, and pizza, and even Dutch apple pie) but still no action down on the Bayou. Fortunately, I've made friends with a nurse practititioner who is also a Brooklyn guy, and he is nice enough to give me a quick examination, call down to my doctor in surgery, and spring me. I offer to e-mail a photo of my next bowel movement.

There are some really tough moments too. I wake up Thursday at 4AM and suddenly burst into tears for about half an hour, then again at 6AM. On Friday I try as hard as I can to comfort a woman who's daughter had just checked in a few rooms down from me. She seemed to be in a place beyond which comfort just couldn't reach. I try to make the most of my time on the 15th floor, but I don't ever ever ever want to go back there again.

My wounds heal rapidly. I'd decided to give myself a year to make some sort of sense of this experience, and I'm still within that time frame and working hard at it. I think it may take even longer, but that's cool too.

Sometime this week I'll get the pathology report back from the lab and I'll know exactly what it was that I had. I'm not expecting any surprises, but by now I'm well-trained enough to expect nothing and everything. In another three months I go back to my oncologist for another check-up. I find my inspiration from, of all people, the writer E.L.Doctorow, who once described writing as a process similar to driving at night. Even though you can only see a short distance ahead, it's incredible how far you can travel in a night. I very much see my battle with illness this way.

In any event, as of today, I am cancer-free again. In April I go back for my next check-up, and hopefully I'll be fine.

Our final score: Solomon 2, Lymphoma 0.

But wait.....there's a penalty flag on the field....

9-0-2-1-Oil

Luke has just finished reciting the Four Questions at our Passover Seder on the Upper East Side. "Why is this night different than all other nights?" he asks. As we set about answering him from our Passover *Haggadahs*, no one suspects that beyond the exclusive consumption of unleavened breads, the ritual washing of hands, and the eating of bitter herbs in remembrance of long-ago slavery in Egypt, the most accurate answer to his question may be this: "On this night, your father will discover that he may have got cancer when he attended Beverly Hills High School thirty years ago." The idea is precipitated by a phone call from my elder sister Lisa in Los Angeles.

"Erin Brockovich is suing Beverly High because the alumni got cancer from the oil wells," my sister says.

My sister is not the kind of person to say "hello" at the beginning of a phone conversation, so it usually takes me a moment to establish context before I can focus on what she's saying.

"Sure she is," I reply. "What are you talking about?"

"I just saw it on TV, Mike," she says. "There are all these kids who are sick."

"You mean the real Erin Brockovich? I ask. "As in, the movie?"

"Yeah. You need to find out what's going on."

Back in 1974 my father accepted a job at the May Company department store in L.A. and moved us to a Spanish colonial house in Beverly Hills. We lived in the poorer section of Beverly Hills –if such a thing can be imagined – about a mile west of Rodeo Drive, and about three million dollars south of where all the movie stars lived. I knew I was too small to play football but I was a fourteen-year-old transfer student and I desperately needed a way to make friends. So for the next two years, with a thick Brooklyn accent and a feeble grip on the ladder of social acceptance, I did my best to get along.

When I was at Beverly High, there were – of all things – two working oil wells right next to the athletic field – a pair of silvery green "grasshoppers" tirelessly pumping out liquid riches from below and subjecting we students to harmless, though cringe-producing comparisons to the Clampett family of *Beverly Hillbillies* fame. For a new student like me, this ostentatious display had particular resonance, and seemed to confirm the notion that my life had now passed from the sublime to the ridiculous.

While I used to see the wells as evidence of, if anything, a sort of "moral" cancer, the idea that they had caused literal cancers seems preposterous. How could I and the other sick alumni have inhaled the seeds of our ruin so long ago, in the safest place any of us had probably ever lived?

When I get home from Passover *seder* I do a quick search and find that the city of Beverly Hills and the oil companies that ran the wells on campus are now facing a massive lawsuit over an alleged "cancer cluster" among the alumni, presumably caused by the oil and gas operations at the school. Upwards of five hundred former students of Beverly Hills High School suspect their cancers and auto-immune disorders may be the result of exposure to toxic gas "constituents," such as benzene and n-hexane, emitting from the oil and natural gas facilities at Beverly High. The suits are being spearheaded by the dynamic duo of environmental law, attorney Edward Masry and his firm's director of environmental research Erin

Brockovich, in what has already become an emotionally pitched and highly public battle.

The next day I call their law firm in southern California. A flood of nervous energy pours through me as I listen to the details of the lawsuit on the phone. Even as I absorb the litany of accusations about lax monitoring and official denials that typify toxic tort litigation, my curiosity about the suit, and my potential involvement therein are tempered by a nagging ambivalence about what I hope to find out. If it were true that somehow the wells had leaked toxic constituents into the air around the track, and if this did indeed correlate to my illness, would I be happy? Relieved? Angry? Cancer has a funny way of forcing you to accept your mortality, and once this acceptance has taken hold it's difficult to return to the murky, psychic terrain of blame. Survival depends upon a certain degree of acceptance, self-forgiveness, and banishment of self-pity, and for now, I'm a survivor. Cancer has been good and bad to me, especially I suppose because I'm lucky enough to be around to ponder it.

It's like in the Passover story, when the Jews were finally freed by Pharaoh, they were left to wander the desert for forty years. The older members of the tribe were gone long before anyone reached the Promised Land. The price of their freedom was in part the reluctant acceptance that their lives were a puzzling mixture of self-knowledge, doubt, and insufficient vindication. And as much as I want to know the truth about how lymphoma found its way inside me, I'm aware of how that truth has already re-ignited my feelings of vulnerability from childhood. Even if I am someone whose destiny was secretly etched long before I was conscious enough to see past the chalk-marked finish line of my youthful dreams (I ran track and played football at Beverly High), my internal cancer *Haggadah* reminds me never to feel sorry for myself. I want to know the truth about the oil wells, but at the same time, I'm afraid of it overtaking the psychological peace I've made with my illness.

That night I pace from one end of my apartment to the other. Next thing I know I'm playfully mimicking the giant strides of my former track event, the high hurdles. I remember how nervous I'd be before the start of each race. Back then I thought the cure for fear was the elimination of fear. But now I know better. The cure is courage in the face of fear. So the next day, armed with this idea, I decide to become a plaintiff in the lawsuit and try to learn the truth.

Though I've never worked as a journalist, I decide to do my own investigation. I pitch the story to a men's health magazine and they accept, and in short order I'm on a plane out to LA, thirty years after the end of my football career. Here's the story I turn in:

Peter Stockmann: Is there anything abnormal about the present conditions?

Dr. Stockmann: To tell you the truth, Peter, I can't say just at this moment—at all events not tonight. There may be much that is very abnormal about the present conditions— and it is possible there may be nothing abnormal about them at all. It is quite possible it may be merely my imagination.

- "An Enemy of the People" by Henryk Ibsen

Science caught up to me twice on the football field at Beverly High. The first time was when I tried to tackle a two-hundred-fifty-pound fullback from our rivals at Mira Costa High School. I was exactly half his weight, and in spite of my little-guy toughness, I found myself lying prone on the field a full three yards back from the spot where I'd endeavored to hit him. My head rang from the force of our impact, and his footsteps sounded like horse's hooves as he raced past me towards the end zone. The lesson I drew from this unhappy collision was that physics trumps determination every time, and the reward for my discovery was that I would never again play middle linebacker for Beverly High. As I stumbled woozily to the sideline, Coach Bushman tried gamely to comfort me. "Shake it off, Solomon," he said gently. "And goddamnit, *never* hit a guy that big above the waist."

My second, inopportune encounter with science is an order of magnitude less predictable.

Stretched along South Moreno Drive, Beverly High has a student-run TV and radio station, a planetarium, three theaters, and an indoor facility known as the "Swim Gym" featuring a basketball court that retracts at the push of a button into a swimming pool. BHHS has a reputation for academic excellence, and it is especially proud of its dramatic arts program, which has yielded a litany of homegrown stars among the alumni: Nicholas Cage, Gina Gershon, and Richard Dreyfuss to name a few. Yet beyond its physical attributes and famous pedigree, the school is a source of pride in its community, a feather in the cap of the public school system as a whole and a testament to the good life and security that await those lucky enough to raise their children here. My mother used to say that "rich or poor, it's better to be rich," and Beverly Hills, I can attest, is no exception to this folksy maxim. Thus on some magnanimous level the very fact of a *public* school serves an additional democratizing role among the elite, leveling the playing field as it were between the well-off, the wealthy and the super wealthy.

At a coffee shop along swanky Beverly Drive, I meet a pretty blond-haired girl named Lori Moss. Now twenty-eight, Moss, began her secondary education at Beverly Hills High School in September of 1978, where she made a passel of good friends and hitched up with a steady boyfriend whom she loved and who adored her. Lori's high school years were the best time in her young life, she tells me, and seemed to portend a bright future. She was smart, confident, and filled with optimism.

But three years after graduation, Lori found out she had Hodgkin's disease, a scary but curable cancer of the lymphatic system. She endured six months of chemotherapy and a month of daily radiation in order to beat the disease into remission, where it remained for seven years. Then suddenly at age twenty-seven, when she thought the cancer nightmare was well behind her, she felt a lump on her neck, which turned out to be thyroid cancer. This time she underwent surgery to remove her thyroid and then ingested a radioactive therapy pill so potent she had to spend three days in total isolation at a hospital, lest she contaminate anyone else. Like most cancer patients, particularly young ones with no family history of cancer, Lori was at a loss to understand how such bad luck had befallen her twice before the age of thirty.

Shortly after her thyroid diagnosis, she sought out Erin Brockovich at a book signing at the Beverly Hills Public Library, where Brockovich was promoting her own personal growth manifesto entitled *Take it From Me: Life's a Struggle But You Can Win.* Moss had been taken with Brockovich since seeing the movie about her in 1992 and reading her book, and she waited patiently for well over an hour to meet her heroine.

"I'm a talker," Brockovich later tells me, with characteristic folksiness. Brockovich is quite a looker too, and the whole push-up bra thing is not a Hollywood invention, not that I notice because I'm here as a journalist.

"Lori told me she'd had the Hodgkin's and then she found out she had thyroid and I thought 'Oh my gosh.' She's a beautiful young girl. I was very taken by her. I asked her where she grew up and she made a comment that she went to Beverly Hills High. I really didn't think anything of it other than I admired this young girl. She had a really great outlook on life and I told her I really didn't know a thing about Beverly Hills High but if I ever learned of anything, I'd call her. I never thought another thing of it."

Several months after she and Moss met, Brockovich was working on a controversial case involving the building of a school atop a methane field in Belmont, California when someone (whom she refuses to identify, citing attorney-client privilege) made a comment to the effect that "if you think Belmont is bad, you should check out what's going on at Beverly Hills High."

Brockovich immediately got back in touch with Moss, who by then had been in contact with two other Beverly High alumni with her same cancers. Brockovich then began — as is her wont — to search the Internet and request documents under the Freedom of Information Act. She discovered that in 1959, the Beverly Hills School Board began accepting bids from several oil companies, whereupon four wells were drilled directly on high school property. Two wells were clearly in evidence just next to the girl's athletic field (the ones I recalled, which pre-date Moss' enrollment). Five years later, a major oil field extending out from the school and known as the East Beverly Hills Oil Field was discovered by Standard Oil and Occidental Petroleum, which led to a major expansion and redrilling operation in 1978. Thanks to a technique known as directional drilling, in which drill bits snake through the earth from one central locus, all of the work was sent underground, save for one visible eyesore of a derrick. Of a proposed thirty oil wells, fully eighteen were ultimately completed beneath school grounds.

The Los Angeles Basin has been the scene of intensive oil drilling since the end of the Civil War, when wildcatters turned their swords into pickaxes in search of black gold. By 1909, the area between the Santa Ana Mountains and the Pacific Ocean had evolved into a major crude oil refining center. Long before the invention of the automobile, crude oil was converted into kerosene and asphalt, among other products, whose demand was in turn driven by the constant growth of Southern California and the switchover of fuel supplies from coal to the more abundant oil. Once the automobile took hold, a period of explosive drilling erupted so that by 1923, fully 20% of the world's total production of crude oil came from the Los Angeles Basin.

It wasn't until Brockovich found the first document to raise her hackles, or as she describes it, "to hack me off," that her investigation gained any forward momentum. The document was an EPA newsletter, known as an "oil spill program update" and dated April 2001, which discussed "creative facades" the industry had adopted to "mask oil operations amid the glamour of Beverly Hills." The reference was to an obscure art project on the Beverly High campus completed in September 2000, which bears with it an irony that is both emblematic and absurd, and which lies very much at the heart of why this case has become such a crusade for Masry and Brockovich.

At a height of one hundred sixty five feet and four inches, the Tower of Hope is "the largest monument in the Western United States" according to the website of Portraits of Hope, the organization that pulled together some 3,000 children to decorate the tower's vinyl panels in a bright, four-sided floral pattern representing the four seasons. These were no ordinary young artists – they were all suffering from serious illnesses ranging from spinal injuries, to burn trauma, to cancer. The Tower is itself an unusual structure, visible from nearly a mile away, and totally at odds with the adjacent gray monoliths of Century City. It resembles in its vertical boxiness a sort of narrow and gleefully gift-wrapped pyramid seemingly left behind by aliens from the planet Hippie. But hidden beneath this improbable shroud is the oil derrick at the center of the Venoco Oil companies operations at Beverly Hills High School – a total of 18 underground wells stretching through the Earth's tectonic plates.

Venoco (pronounced, VEH-no-co), which assumed control of the leases in April 1995, is only the latest in a series of oil companies at Beverly Hills High School. As all of the plaintiffs in the lawsuits attended Beverly High between 1975 and 1996, one of the key issues in any forthcoming litigation will be who is liable for damages, if any.

I drive out to the law offices of Masry & Vititoe, at the edge of the San Fernando Valley, where US Highway 101 grows so wide there's actually a sign that reads: *Ventura Freeway – Four Left Lanes.* The hills abutting the valley are an exquisite mix of earth tones – brown and green hillocks peppered with yellow flowers, like a vast Impressionist canvas. The law firm is located in a non-descript business park in the town of Westlake Village, with an atrium so brand new that by contrast its furnishings – shiny cloisonné pottery, state flags and *faux* gilded furniture – strike me as what a Museum of a Law Office might someday look like.

Brockovich and Masry had already submitted their first twenty-five administrative claims in the case, a legal precursor to the lawsuits. Unlike a class-action suit, in which every plaintiff shares the same cause and outcome, these suits are a series of direct actions, organized by specific illnesses but focused primarily on four types of cancers – Hodgkin's disease, non-Hodgkin's lymphoma, testicular cancer, and thyroid cancer, in addition to several auto-immune disorders.

Edward Masry (whom Albert Finney played so memorably in the movie) leads me past a long line of windowed offices and a wall bearing framed movie posters from the only film that really matters much out here. He greets me as a client and a journalist – neither he nor I is quite sure what to make of me. At seventy years old, Masry is imbued with the type of youthful vigor and bluster that accompanies a lifetime of facing down opponents larger than he. I quickly learn that he and I are scatological soulmates. Says Masry:

"This is just a big cover up. It's all bullshit. But we expect that from the government, we fight this all the time. What's important is, what's that jury gonna do? And the way it looks right now, when that jury finds out the lengths that this school district and AQMD (South Coast Air Quality Management District) went to try to cover up what was going on, they're not gonna be happy. Cause they've got kids in school. You know, the school district keeps digging itself a bigger hole. I hope they keep doing this testing that's not valid compared to ours."

Masry's air-quality testing, furtively conducted on school grounds by the firm's environmental specialist Jim Drury, came up with concentrations of benzene – a known carcinogen – measuring 56 micrograms per meter in the air around the high school – some 28 times higher than the average background concentrations reported by the Environmental Protection Agency for Los Angeles County. These readings carry with them an associated cancer risk 1600 times higher than the AQMD's "maximum acceptable risk" for schools of one in a million. These are the kind of numbers that would have bristled the hair of the anti-environmentalist James Watt; to the city of Beverly Hills, and the AQMD, they were practically an act of war.

"Do you think I'm an idiot?" Masry says, when I ask him about Barry Wallerstein, a Beverly High alumnus who happens to be the current executive officer of the South Coast AQMD, and who in that official capacity has asserted that Masry's data may be tainted by a lapse in its chain of custody. "When Erin came to me with her feelings that there was something going on there, my first reaction was 'we're going to attack the city of Beverly Hills? And the school district? We better make sure of what we're doing. This is going to be a major story if this thing breaks.'"

No stranger to tactics, nor to ensuring that a story breaks, Masry began to leak his findings to a local TV station, KCBS-LA, which in turn contacted Wallerstein and asked if he'd be willing to conduct his own testing on camera. Wallerstein demurred, and instead dispatched AQMD inspectors on a series of air sampling missions in and around the high school, where they found no abnormal levels whatsoever. Drury, who proudly tells me of being thrown off the BHHS campus three times as he chained Summa air sampling canisters to various spots around the athletic fields, disputes these results, and maintains that his readings were accurate, and in Masry's words, "admissible as evidence in any court in the United States." Yet Wallerstein remains skeptical: "We didn't find anything out of the normal with the benzene level, which is the pollutant of major concern here related to cancer. Bottom line is, we can't explain how the Masry firm came up with the higher benzene levels."

Wallerstein says Venoco "voluntarily" shut down operations when first contacted by AQMD, and then resumed production upon the release of AQMD's first report indicating no abnormalities in the air quality around the facility. However, AQMD forced production to a halt again when it refused to issue a permit for a piece of Venoco's natural gas venting equipment due to excessive benzene readings. These readings, still, were well below the toxic nightmare Drury claimed to have found.

I call Mike Edwards, Venoco's vice-president, who believes the public is unjustifiably alarmed, owing to a lack of understanding about oil development. "I have talked to a lot of parents and I think the test results give us some comfort because we're around oil and gas operations and we understand it. When you look out over the ball field, you see kids on the basketball court, you see kids on the softball field, you see people out at the track, you realize parents are going to want more information. We've always said we'll continue to cooperate to try to get them the answers that they want."

The other half of the equation in the case is the epidemiological underpinning of the cancers and autoimmune diseases, such as hemolytic anemia and Hashimoto's (thyroid) disease, that have been reported by the alumni. Whether or not air quality is ultimately determined to be a factor, incidences of disease as high as those reported by Masry & Vititoe are well outside of the parameters one might normally expect to find. The number of illnesses reported has steadily increased right up to the time of this writing, with non-Hodgkins lymphomas, for one, being reported at a rate four times the norm among alumni.

Wendy Cozen, a toxicology professor at the University of Southern California (USC) who has quickly become the "Erin Brockovich of the defense" in the time since the allegations were first made public, issued a report saying that cancer levels among Beverly Hills residents, while at the "upper limits of normal," are nonetheless symptomatic only of elevated cancer rates in Los Angeles in general. Cozen's only concession to the charges is her opinion that thyroid cancers are deserving of further study, but only because they're at elevated levels in Los Angeles as a whole.

"That's not the issue," says Masry. "We're not talking about the city of Beverly Hills. We're talking about the alumni of Beverly Hills High School. Most of our clients don't live in Beverly Hills."

Surprisingly, or rather, stunningly when one considers that most of the plaintiffs no longer live in Beverly Hills, there has been no direct outreach to Beverly High alumni by either the city or the school district. Lori Moss, for one, lives several miles away in Westwood. I, for another, only heard about the case because my sister saw it on KCBS-TV when she was visiting Los Angeles over Passover. The BHHS Alumni Association tells me that they lack the means to send out notice to the roughly 15,000 addresses on their present roll, but when I press and ask if perhaps they'd included a mention of the case in either this year's 75th school anniversary mailing notice or the annual fundraising letter, I'm told that this "is just not one of our functions."

Though Beverly Hills is a community not generally known for its aversion to displays of wealth, money has, ironically, received little mention by either side as a motivating factor in the case thus far. Oil royalties to the Beverly Hills Unified School District (BHUSD), according to its besieged supervisor Dr. Gwen Gross, approach $300,000 annually. In addition, homeowners within the surface area of the oil fields collect royalty checks that hover around $200 a year, depending on overall oil revenues and prices, although Carolyn Spiegel, a twenty-five year resident of South Roxbury Drive whom I met, received a check one year for over $15,000. While Spiegel's royalty payments are fairly atypical of the several hundred private leaseholders above the Eastern oilfield, she is typical of the parents and residents I meet in that she's been following the news closely and says she is satisfied –for now – with the AQMD reports and Wendy Cozen's assurances that nothing is wrong. After she jokingly admits to being suspicious of me just "walking" down the street (I am the only pedestrian in sight, in spite of the fulsome sidewalks), I identify myself as the boy who used to live three houses away and she graciously invites me into her house. "My best friend at Beverly used to live here," I tell her, and later I decide to reveal that: "I'm one of the 'kids' with cancer." There is unfortunately no gracious way to say the latter, and my confession seems to suddenly prompt her daughter Edana into a remembrance of a girl with a thyroid problem two blocks away. It is hard not to read anything into Edana's unscientific revelation – harder still to ignore the sense that people are more worried than they want to admit.

The closest Brokovich has come to a "smoking gun" is a 1978 Environmental Impact Report prepared for the city of Beverly Hills at the time that the directional drilling and a pursuant modification of city code to allow it were proposed. The EIR asks a series of multiple choice questions, which can be answered "yes," "no," or "maybe." While the majority of questions address issues of aesthetics, noise, and groundwater impact (a focus which infuriates Brockovich), question 17 asks:

Will the proposal result in:

a)   *Creation of any health hazard or potential health hazard (excluding mental health)?*

b)   *Exposure of people to potential health hazards?*

In each case the answer checked is "maybe."

Judging from the conflicting epidemiological and air quality data, it is a long way from these "maybes" to a confirmed correlation between cancer and oil and gas production at the high school, though the lack of follow-up monitoring of on-site air quality over the past 25 years is, if nothing else, unsettling. According to Wallerstein, there are over 28,000 industrial facilities under the jurisdiction of South Coast AQMD, which are monitored by seven primary stations and thirty-two substations throughout the L.A. Basin. Unless specific complaints are received, air quality is monitored through this type of "representative" readings.

Both Cozen at USC, and another toxicologist I speak with at UC Berkeley, Professor Martyn Smith, affirm that Hodgkin's disease, for one, has no known correlation with benzene exposure. Non-Hodgkin's lymphoma on the other hand, is the subject of debate amongst toxicologists, according to Smith, who goes so far as to call a correlation between the two "highly probable."

Masry is philosophical about his approach.

"I think when you say Beverly Hills High, and a toxic dump, you're going to have a lot of people that'll say 'that's impossible'. We're not talking Shitville; we're talking an affluent community with a lot of doctors and lawyers; they wouldn't permit it to happen. But the vast majority of that community had no idea what was underground. If that had been above ground, it'd be a different story. Those parents would've been down there and it would've been shut before it ever opened. They didn't know what was going on. Let me put it this way, if this were in a minority area, it'd be shut, because in minority areas they don't trust the government. Beverly Hills is a different animal."

For both the credulous and the skeptical (and those like me, who are a little of both), the allegations about what may or may not have happened to the alumni of Beverly Hills High School can't help but raise even larger, more disturbing questions about the assumptions we make about industry and public health. Illness does not discriminate between the well-heeled and the needy, and thus what's really at issue is not just that society's ears tend to prick up in response to a case of such high-profile – enveloped as it is by the luster of wealth and celebrity – but rather that many of the comforting reassurances we allow ourselves about the public trust may be more willful than we care to acknowledge.

Masry and Brockovich held their first public meeting to discuss the case at the Beverly Hills Hotel. They laid out their findings to an audience of some seven hundred people made up mostly of local residents and sick people. Lori Moss described a shouting match that seemed to capture not only the tone of the evening, but also the tenor of the entire case thus far.

"One guy got up and said: 'Well what about my property value?' And a girl got up and said: 'Fuck your property value. I'm thirty years old and I have breast cancer.'"

It is hard not to be swayed by such naked suffering, even when the relevance of breast cancer to this case is still highly in dispute. In a town like Beverly Hills, where ideals of public safety and protection are the nerve and fiber of the social contract, people are slow to embrace such a staggering assault on the material and psychic infrastructure. But for folks like me, who still wrestle the demons of an uncertain future and perhaps an even more uncertain past, it is difficult to overlook the understated observation that Martyn Smith shares with me at the end of our conversation:

"It's probably not a good idea to put a high school on top of an oil well."

Standing Room Only

The past is never dead. It isn't even past.

-William Faulkner

As time passes, I begin to change. When I finally quit smoking years ago, the urge to reach for a cigarette slowly dissipated from every minute, to every hour, to every day, until eventually entire months would go by without me thinking about smoking. Cancer follows a similar mental trajectory, at least for me. Even though this is a story about survival, not everyone makes it.

Stephen J. Gould, whose brilliant ideas about the origins of man illuminated his generation and many to follow, and whose mathematical acumen bailed me out of a deep and fearful funk, dies. He fought off mesothelioma only to succumb to another type of cancer entirely. My sweet friend St. Clair survives his tumor but loses his battle to a pulmonary embolism. I begin going to the obituaries again to see which other glowing spirit has been sent packing from this cold and heartless world. And I wonder: how many other times has my own number been up, only to be snatched from the jaws of death by some matter of inches, or seconds, or happenstance?

When I was a baby I suddenly and inexplicably dehydrated and the doctors were almost unable to find a vein on my tiny body through which to inject me with the fluids I desperately needed. They wound up injecting me in the head and saving my infant life.

When I was sixteen I flew out of the driver's seat and onto the floor of my friend's Dodge Van at the entrance to the Golden Gate Bridge.

We were going forty miles an hour. Our vehicle spun around several times across five lanes of traffic before coming to a halt six inches in front of a brick wall. But because it was long after midnight, the road was deserted and hence my life and that of my friend's was spared. Any other time of day and we were scrap metal.

At twenty-five I dove awkwardly into the churning waters off the coast of Hawaii, slammed my hip on lava rocks, and miraculously avoided slamming my head as well. I came up gasping for air, clutching my hip, and realizing then and there that the breath I sucked in so heartily was a gift I didn't necessarily deserve.

How many other times have I almost died? What about all the times I was at great risk and never even knew it (for instance, where exactly am I each time a drunk driver falls asleep at the wheel?)? I ask that because my "experience" with cancer has been so surreal that I often feel as if it never really happened. As if the danger was never any greater than when I dehydrated, or the van was spinning, or the tide was sucking me onto the prehistoric surface of the land of Aloha (a word that, fittingly, means both "hello" and "goodbye").

Back in New York my nine-month check-up arrives and as I slink down East 67th Street towards the hospital, I tell myself that the third time's a charm. Anything to dissipate the fear of another fight in Round Three. This time I come up lucky. I am still cancer-free. Another nine months go by and again my tests come up clean. So Portlock puts me on a once-a-year testing regimen and each time I come and go with a clean bill of health.

I have, in spite of all my fear and surgery, effectively dodged a bullet. I've lived to tell the tale. Isn't that ultimately the best measure of all that's gone on in my life? Well, I don't want to bad mouth survival, but the answer I believe is a resounding "no." Surviving isn't enough, although hell, it's a good beginning. When I am long gone, under the ground, up in the clouds, or wherever it is one goes (Oberammergau? Mars?) there will be ample time to hail my survival of yesteryear. Matter of fact, I would like to suggest that a good deal of said hailing take place at my funeral, as I've always hoped it would be a devastatingly sad yet somehow uplifting event that might merit a full-page mention in a national newspaper, say, or on a highly trafficked website. Unlike what anyone else wants, I trust.

I got lucky. I know many people now who are, in my view, massively unlucky. Tormented by cancer or some other horrific disease. Tortured by themselves. Hopeless and beaten-down and angry. All I can say to a person in that awful situation is that I am just beginning to learn to understand what you are up against. I am like the petty little apprentice collecting coals for the fires of Hell. I've felt the heat but have thus far been spared the full force of the burning.

I hope that some of what worked for me – laughing, crying, taking notes, selling tickets to my intestinal Mardi Gras – might someday work for someone else, even though we get so fucked over at times it is hard to feel much more than just alone and numb. Besides, if my doctors had been any less excellent, I might be laughing and crying all the way to the undertaker. So I just try to keep moving forward.

Luke and I tough it out in the tiny apartment for the next two years. What we lack in living space we try to make up for in fun, and the forced proximity of the place causes us to grow even closer. Layla and I arrange a joint custody schedule whereby he spends a week with me followed by a week with her, and while it can sometimes be the best of both worlds, it is also sometimes the worst of both worlds. I miss Luke so much when he's not there. But we both love our kid, and he loves both of us, so this is about the best we feel we can do by him and by ourselves.

Eventually I try dating again, and after sixteen years of being in a relationship, it's pretty much a disaster. I want to date women close to me in age but at my age, all those women want to do is get married and have kids. New York suddenly reverberates with the sound of ticking biological clocks. I don't blame the women I meet for wanting what they want, and honestly, I would love more children myself but I've got a few things to sort out, okay?

Well, actually, not okay, comes their collective response. One woman goes so far as to tell me that I'm so terrified of relationships that I've become, in her words, a "walking condom." On top of this, every time I even meet someone I like I start to think about when and how I'm ever going to tell them I've got all this baggage: cancer, divorce, a teetering career. Oh and by the way I'm not ready for a relationship either. Maybe I should get them really drunk and just blurt it out, I think. Or maybe I should just get really drunk myself and forget about the whole idea of ever getting laid again.

I go through the motions, and happily, all the women I meet seem pretty cool about me having cancer, though of course I don't *currently* have cancer so that probably helps some. I have a couple dalliances that go nowhere. And then like an idiot I fall in love with a stunning woman close to me in age, who wants to get married and have kids. We meet cute, at least what passes for cute in my world. Her name is Natalie and she's also a documentary filmmaker. I meet her at a film market we're both attending, where we're both hoping to raise money to finish our respective movies. Her film is about her father, a gambling addict who disappeared into the streets of Las Vegas.

She doesn't seem very enamored of me at first. She's barely tolerating me, honestly. But I'm persistent (fortune favors the bold, they say) and at one point I ask her: "Is this how you make your entire living? Doing documentaries?" It's pretty much a rhetorical question in the documentary world. Very few of us are able to survive solely on the skimpy-if-any salaries of documentary filmmaking, and Natalie's no exception. She tells me she's also an actress, and matter of fact, she just came from another film festival up in Woodstock where a film in which she stars was premiering. "Who's the director?" I ask. "Oh, you wouldn't know him, " she says. It turns out I know a lot of the most obscure film directors you can imagine, I say, thanks to that gig I used to have at the Italian film festival. And by the way, I'm separated from my wife and I have cancer.

Except I only think about saying the last part, then decide to wait it out. Natalie says: "The director's name is John O'Brien."

Suddenly I sense an opportunity I'd never have been able to foresee. His name is music to my ears.

"John O'Brien?" I say. "The sheep farmer from Vermont?"

"You know him?" she says, skeptically.

"Not only do I know him. I kiss my ex-wife in his second movie. I was an extra."

And it's true. John grew up and still lives on a sheep farm in Vermont, though he's more a Harvard-educated gentleman farmer than a bona fide sheep farmer. We became friends a decade earlier when I selected one of his films to be in the film festival. He invited Layla and me up to visit and we wound up going to Vermont right when he was shooting his third film, *Vermont is for Lovers.* Layla and I were assigned to sit in the audience during the wedding scene, and as the bride and groom whisk up the aisle past us, we kiss. Not exactly the kind of thing you think will one day be an icebreaker with another woman, but life can be funny that way.

In short order Natalie and I start dating, and things are great for a few weeks, but then Natalie wants to know if I'm willing to eventually get serious and take our relationship to the next step. Even though

I've filed for divorce with Layla, and even though I'm already fed up with the whole dating scene (it just seems to have grown weirder for me in the interim, or else I'm just weirder) I'm still totally paranoid about getting back into a serious relationship. So I resist. About a month later I move Luke and myself into a small loft about a half a block away from where Layla lives. The loft has an open floor plan with no rooms yet, only a small curtained off area, where I decide to place Luke's bedroom. Conspicuously absent is another bedroom that I might eventually share with a woman (read: Nat) were we to get into a serious relationship. I tell Nat that I'll eventually build a couple of proper bedrooms in the loft but since she and I are only just dating what's the rush? I'm still not comfortable with her sleeping over except when Luke is staying over at Layla's.

Besides, who needs physical walls when my psychological walls are so clearly impenetrable? Of course I don't say anything like this to Nat, nor do I possess the kind of self-awareness necessary to know it's even going on with me, but to Nat it's as if I've drawn a line in the sand.

A half a year goes by and then Natalie tells me there's a guy who's been interested in her for months, and he's ready to get married and have kids if things work out, so if I'm really sure things are not headed anywhere serious between us then she'd like to remain friends but move on romantically. I say sure, and thank her for her candor. We officially break up.

Mission accomplished. I've successfully fended off the challenge to my freedom, and autonomy, and single Dad-ness. And as a result, I am now free and happy to take on whatever new challenges life offers me.

Only I'm totally miserable. Profoundly miserable, and angry as all get out. I'm angry that some guy has been snooping around my girlfriend, and I'm angry that Nat could be so calculating about what she wants. She's going to start dating a guy she barely knows because he might want to have a future with her and get married?? I can't believe anyone would think that way. Aren't you supposed to be deeply attracted to each other? Aren't you supposed to first find out if you could even fall in love before you talk about marriage and kids?

Of course it never dawns on me that I'm in love with Nat and even though I've said I would love to have more children I've firmly ruled out the idea of getting married again. So I call Nat and tell her that I'm willing to give it a try if we can just slow down the pace a bit. I suggest we try living together first, to at least see how we do with that, and if that works then we can see eventually about marriage. But she says no, and tells me that she's decided we shouldn't speak to each other for the next six months because it's too painful and it's the only way she's going to be able to move past me and get on with what she truly wants.

I don't know what I want. I mean, I know I want Nat to stop dating this other guy, in part because I think it's skewing her vision of what's going on with us (not to mention my vision....I'm jealous but at the same time incredulous about the whole thing. The guy sounds like some kind of lifetime lonely heart, probably for good reason I assume, snort, chide and snicker to myself.) And I want Nat to just wait until I am ready for us to have a real future together, even though I can't imagine that ever happening because I'm so jaded about marriage. I even try to coax more time from Nat by telling her how Layla and I dated for two years, then moved in together for two more before we wound up getting married (as if that were some recipe for successful marriage, which clearly it is not). But the truth is, no matter how I try to present it, in terms of wanting a relationship, she's on a bullet train and I'm on Thomas the Tank Engine.

So I give up. And I cry a lot. And I bemoan the cruelty of not enough time to heal, and refresh, and bloom anew.

And then a week later Nat calls. She's been really sad, she says, and she realizes she's still in love with me. We agree to get together and talk and the instant I see her I know that somehow I've got to find a way to hang on to this woman. So I say the two words I probably should have just said from Day One, because they are always true when you feel you've met someone special:

I'm open.

Epilogue

Two years later Nat and I take a cab to City Hall and get married. And then at long last we move in together. And then four years later, after an ordeal that rivals cancer survival in its ability to turn people's lives upside down (but alas, that's probably another book) we adopt a beautiful young boy from birth and name him Gabriel. He is nothing short of a dream come true.

After eight years of trying to make a movie with no money, Joe and I eventually finish the Melvin Van Peebles documentary, thanks to an angel investor named Kiki who Joe reconnects with from his high school days, and our movie *How to Eat Your Watermelon in White Company (and Enjoy It)* gets released in New York and about eight other cities around the country. Natalie finishes her movie too.

And just like that life goes on. Luke lives with us every other week, but now he's got a little brother he adores and who adores him. He writes poetry, plays guitar and says one day he wants to become a writer and a filmmaker.

I spend a lot of my time searching for a deeper meaning to the unexpected travails of my life. "Why me?" in certain instances. "Why not me?" in others. I aspire to a type of future whereby something of what I know now can benefit another human being: my sons, my neighbor's son, maybe the son or daughter of a person I will never even meet. I haven't mentioned an epitaph for my tombstone yet, but I wouldn't mind something along the lines of "He Didn't Only Take From This World."

I try to measure my life in density instead of distance, even though I'm still a big fan of distance. Huge fan, actually. Still, I ask myself how much of my fear did I cast aside? What depths did I manage to rise up from? How much light did I manage to throw upon the dark walls of hopelessness?

If you actually do wind up making it to my funeral, feel free to ask those questions about me. Answer them as honestly as you wish. I can take it. Take a poll among the multitudes that will almost certainly be gathered there and solicit their opinions if you like.

No matter what answers you come up with, I will still ask for one small indulgence. Please be gentle. There are a couple of kids in the crowd who want to hear nice things about their Dad. Or – if my luck's held out – maybe those kids are grown men now, looking out at their own kids and trying to think of something meaningful to tell them at a time like this. Perhaps that the horrible struggles inside our minds and bodies can build strength instead of despair, in spite of all the evidence to the contrary. If so, and if you can find it in your heart to leave them and their brood with this small seed of hope – even if it defies all logic and reason to do so – I would really appreciate it.

Otherwise, I may be forced to rethink my entire funeral.

Acknowledgments

During the writing of this book, I became deeply indebted to my friends Joe Angio and Gary Van Wyk for their masterful editing skills, and for their boundless compassion and solidarity through some troubled times, both physical and grammatical. I'm also enormously grateful to my friend Liz Szabla for encouraging me to dust this manuscript off and to give it new life, and to Gilly Halpairn for helping me get it out there once finished.

Big love and gratitude to Aaron Cohen, who led by example and who pushed me to go forward, and Srully Wolfson for the space to do it in. Judith Kelman, if the whole world had a writing coach as wonderful and as funny as you, no one would do anything but write. And laugh. Stephanie Marrou, I will never forget all the hours you dedicated to typing up my handwritten notes. *Gracias infinitas* for putting up with me at my literal, or rather, illegible worst. Steven Varni, your cogent insights as I reached the home stretch are eclipsed in importance only by the extreme grace with which you offered them. Many thanks are also due Miranda Beeson and Peter Cameron for helping an unknown nobody navigate a big world of Books.

Chris Liebertz thank you for your kind words of support and encouragement.

Lisa, my darling older sister, no one has inspired me to write for as long or as devoutly as you have. There is no true measure of the value of that belief in me.

As this is a book about a personal struggle, I want to acknowledge my eternal gratitude to my remarkable doctors and nurses for keeping me alive, and for rescuing my spirits from their various and sundry plummets. The simplest tribute to you is this: No you, No me.

Owing to some reputations that may — ahem - need protecting, I haven't used everyone's real names in this book, so I'd like to collectively thank my friends here by saying that I don't know how the hell I got so lucky in friendship but I can't think of it without tears welling up in my eyes. Now it's indeed funny...but you were there for me when I was living in a run-down psychological shanty on the outskirts of Bummer City. Thanks especially to Steven, my oracle, for teaching me how to fight.

Collette Stephens, Sharon Thomas, and Elena Quadrani sweated it all out with me and my family and bailed water when our ship was listing. Mom and Dad, you somehow hung in there throughout, and because of you I always felt I had someone to catch me if I fell too far. When they were giving out parents, it's clear I got cuts in line. I'm also forever thankful to Sue Phillips for her unflagging love and support and to my kid sister Romy for always being so sweet to me. My brother Andrew was and is quite simply the best brother a guy could ever dream of having, and a damned good doctor to boot. Thank you for always showing up for me or finding someone to come up with a good answer to my endless questions.

Luke and Gabriel, I'd need an entire other book to describe what you mean to me. You boys are the music in my soul, for which I'm thankful every day.

Natalie, my loyal and lovely partner, and my compass on Earth, there is nothing more fulfilling about traveling the road of the future than knowing I'll always be traveling it together with you.